Fifteen Surefire Tips for Relieving Back Pain

(Plus 192 Others, Just in Case)

Andrew Scott Kirschner, D.O.

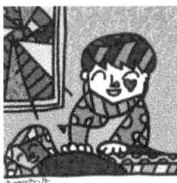

backtogether media

To my love, Donna.

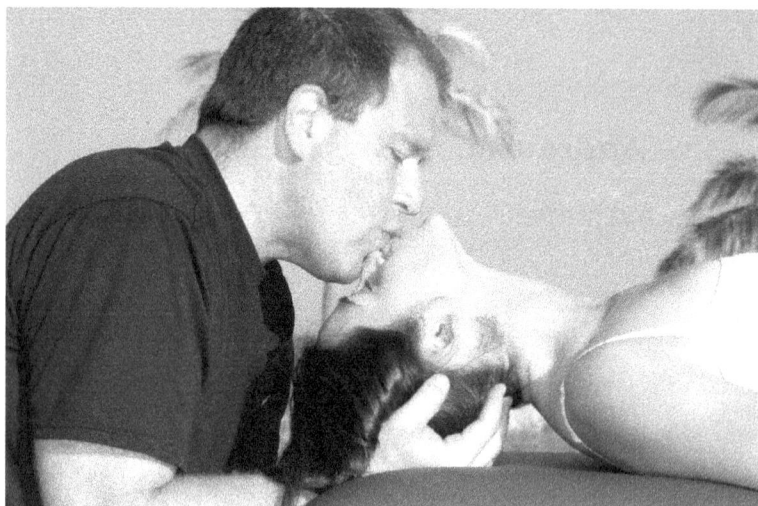

Acknowledgements:

To all my friends and family, too numerous to mention individually: You are the best. I love you all.

Ella & Maya- *You are my inspiration.*

Mom, Dad & Julie- *I always love and appreciate you, even when I act like I don't.*

Galen- *It's all because of you.*

Stan- *Thanks for helping me round out the concept!*

Cliff, Pete & Jorden- You are the BEST.

Fred & Greg- *The cover of this book makes me smile.*

Robin- *You pushed me to write. Thanks!*

Joy- *Formatter extraordinaire.*

Jesse- *Keep up the great work!*

.

Contents

Foreword

Congratulations on taking an important step towards a pain-free lifestyle.

In my line of work, I recommend that people embrace their pain. No, I'm not a professional dominatrix. I teach childbirth -probably one of the only instances in human experience where pain serves a positive function (It's part of a feedback mechanism that makes contractions more efficient). I teach my students to welcome their pain and give them strategies to live with it: deep breathing, relaxation, meditation, acceptance, swaying, etc. But if you are reading this book, you're not likely facing an upcoming labor and your pain is NOT a signal that good things (like a sweet little baby) are coming your way.

Instead, your pain is a perfect signal that something is wrong. In all likelihood, you have a diagnosis of some sort (where your pain originates) and now it's time to make a change.

Luckily, the book you hold in your hands will set you on the path towards reducing --or even eliminating altogether-- pain's ugly grip on your life. Within these pages, Dr. Kirschner clearly explains how pain works in your body and your life. Better still, he'll offer you amazing suggestions as to how to examine your own life --everything from how you're sleeping to how you've organized your kitchen-- and take positive steps towards change.

As a childbirth teacher, I know the extent to which the journey through pain can be internally focused. But the journey away from pain quickly moves from an internal state to an external one. You need to examine what's going on inside your head, your body, your bed, your closet, your car, and every dimension of your daily life to see all of the many places that you can eradicate what Dr. Kirschner rightly calls the "anatomic bombs" that can trip you up. When you've eliminated these obstacles between yourself and a pain-free existence, you'll feel amazing.

I've made my life with Andy for the last eighteen years and I can assure you of his intense, passionate commitment to the cause of helping people eliminate the scourge of back and neck pain from their lives. He has worked tirelessly in his quest to seek out the causes and effective treatment of back and neck pain. He has treated thousands of people in his own clinical practice and has taught other practitioners and lay people worldwide. Over the years, he has developed simple, safe and effective techniques that empower back pain sufferers and their loved ones to reduce and even eliminate their pain. You are in for a treat.

Just a quick note of caution: Breaking patterns takes effort. In the work that you'll do here, Dr. Kirschner will encourage you to take steps, small and large that ask you to really examine your lifestyle from a back-friendly perspective. If you take his steps to heart, you will come to see the world in new ways and, hopefully, come to see yourself as an empowered person, who can take control of your pain. Good luck on your journey towards a back-friendly life.

-Donna Kirschner, PhD.

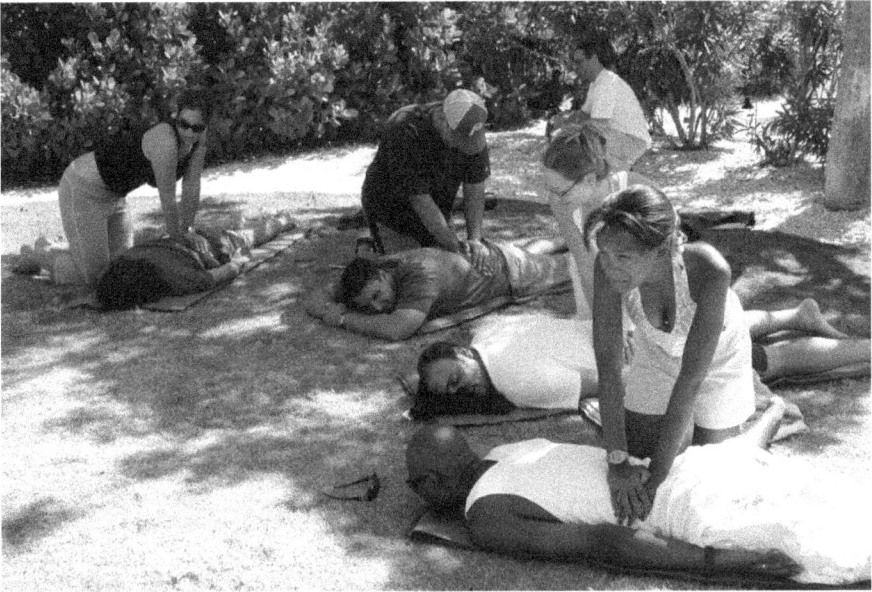

Couples learning hands-on techniques for relieving back pain

at a Back Together Live seminar in Miami, Florida

How to use this book:

Ok, you've picked up this book, so it's probably safe to assume you or someone close to you has back pain. Let's say for a second that you read the title of this book, and you are really impatient, or you're just reading this book in a bookstore with no real intention of buying it, and you just want the 15 back pain relieving tips on my double secret list. I suppose you *could* just jump ahead to my double-secret list and cheat your way to a more back-friendly lifestyle. But really, imagine how cheap and tainted you might feel if you did that! However, if you really want to do things *right*- and find *long-lasting benefits* you should sit down and read the book- the *whole* book. Seriously, it's not that long.

I have worked tirelessly to bring you a great and effective compilation of tips to help relieve your pain and keep it away. As you read through the chapters, consider keeping a small notebook (for which I will give you additional uses). Keep a simple list of the tips and ideas you read that most clearly apply to you. This list will provide a personalized starting point as you navigate your way to the back-pain-free lifestyle.

Before you do anything, speak with your physician. Occasionally, back pain can be the only indication that something serious is going on- perhaps something not even directly related to the spine. Find out the cause of your back pain before you try any of the suggestions in this book. There is absolutely *nothing* in this book that could harm you, but it is critically important to have a diagnosis. This will prevent you from possibly glossing over a potentially serious problem, and furthermore help you to make more educated decisions as you work to create a pain-free life.

As you apply the tips, keep in mind that your pain probably took some time to evolve to the point it's at right now. Give these suggestions some time to work, and little by little, they will.

The names of the individual's in this book have not been changed because honestly, what's the point?

Enjoy!

Part I. The Talk

Introduction

I began my last book by explaining to readers that I simply had no appreciation for the entire genre of self-help books. Many people perceived this as *slightly* ironic given that I made this statement at the beginning of what clearly was, in fact, a self-help book. So with that out of the way, let's be clear about one thing: I still hate self-help books.

This hatred has only become more ironic since the release of that book: *Back Together- Hands on Healing for Couples*. My issue with all of these (*other*) books has been that many authors in this genre profess to have some special knowledge that will ultimately solve whatever problem the book addresses. (Don't get me wrong- there are *some* good self-help books out there- like say for instance -*mine*, but I still feel like most of them are just silly.) It doesn't matter the topic- it could be money, fitness, weight loss- even back pain- many of the authors are self-declared gurus, and those of us on the other end were willing consumer-pupils, ready to absorb their special knowledge (Sometimes their special knowledge wasn't all that special: Wanna lose weight? You should eat less. Really? *Genius*! Even better, I was asked to write a forward for a book that recommended a diet almost exclusively of green vegetables as a cure for pretty much everything. I politely declined.) After the release of my book, I found that all of a sudden *I was the guru*, which was exactly the *opposite* of what I aimed to achieve by writing it in the first place. I started getting letters, emails and calls, all asking for my special knowledge, some believing that perhaps I had a magic spell or incantation that would make their pain vanish. The requests were different from those that a doctor usually gets; it felt as though some folks believed that if I simply placed my hands on their painful spines, then their discomfort would miraculously vanish.

Let me restate this: I am not a guru. I don't have any special knowledge or mystical secret to impart to you which will magically relieve your back pain. I am a physician who has been treating back pain for more than fifteen years. During that time, I've accumulated what I feel to be a pretty good understanding of many of the things that help relieve the pain, and gone to great lengths to weed out those things that don't. I obsessively observe people's body mechanics, how various ergonomic considerations affect them in their daily lives, and how different activities can influence their pain. For the purposes of this (*fabulous*) book, we will focus on those things that will help, which brings me to the main point I am trying to make through all of this: At the end of the day I hope that you will understand the elements that make up the *pain-free lifestyle*, and then you will be the guru, and ultimately that's going to take some of the pressure off of me.

Who is Andy Kirschner anyway?

Why should you care what I have to say about back pain? After all, I just got through telling you that I don't have any magic powers. What separates what I have to offer from everything else out there about back pain?

I've been a physician since 1995, and while I'd always wanted to become a doctor- like my dad, who is a head & neck surgeon- I've always been fascinated with the spine. My first interest in back pain came about when I was fourteen years old, and had the misfortune of seeing my grandfather pass away from pancreatic cancer. The first clue that he had a problem? Yep- you guessed it- *back pain.*

Since that time I have made it a point to understand

everything there is to know about back pain. What causes it, what makes it worse, which treatments work, which ones don't, and how one's habits and lifestyle can make pain better or worse. Back and neck pain are my obsession, and finding ways to make them go away is my profession and passion.

I've been in private practice since 1998, and during that time I have been lucky enough to work with and treat patients from pretty much every walk of life: From people working on assembly lines with heavy machinery to executives with super plush offices. From professional athletes at the peak of physical conditioning to Special Athletes competing with complex physiological challenges. From young children to- wait 'till you hear this- a woman of 102 years old who still takes a 2 mile walk *every day* that there isn't snow on the ground. My point here is that I've seen it all. In treating this amazing and wonderful variety of patients, I've had the opportunity to filter through much of the nonsense, hone in on the things that work, and collect enough clinical and anecdotal evidence to give you information that I know will help you reduce your pain.

I have always believed that the human body is an amazing piece of engineering, with a fantastic ability to heal itself. Conversely, I've noticed that when it doesn't heal itself, it is often because we aren't treating ourselves particularly well -sometimes consciously, other times unconsciously. In my professional life, I've generally worked under the belief that the less you rely on magic potions (i.e.- medications), the better off you will be. The information I want to share with you includes many of the lifestyle modifications I've found to help you avoid dependency on some of these medications, and to help yourself live pain-free.

Why a second book?

"My back pain came back," is a sentence no physician or therapist ever wants to hear. We doctors frequently spend a lot of time trying to help our patients find relief from their back & neck pain- medication, manual medicine, physical therapy, exercise therapy, stretching, massage- we sometimes need to employ the whole gambit of modalities to find the combinations that will finally provide relief. Why don't we want to hear that it came back? Well, the first reason should be self-evident; we feel badly that our patient feels pain. Even doctors with the *worst* bedside manner wish the best for their patients (even if they sometimes have a rough time showing it). Secondly, when we hear that your pain came back, it's a lot like finding out your kid got expelled from school; here you put all this effort and work into something (your child? your back?) and then they *let you down*. I know this may seem a somewhat self-centered concept, but honestly, it's really a terrible feeling, and one that, in my career, I have experienced far too many times. Now, know this: This didn't occur because of my abilities, or those of the people to whom I refer patients, or because I'm dealing with a bunch of non-compliant patients. A host of factors (many of which we will cover in later sections of the book) produce this phenomenon. Consequently, some doctors will try to decrease the likelihood that their patients will experience reoccurrence of their pain by prescribing medications that *ensure* their patients won't hurt- but sometimes this can be to the detriment of the patient.

In my *Back Together* book and program, I provide hands-on modalities, psychological strategies, and rudimentary ergonomic suggestions to help couples to help each other to relieve their pain. I designed the program to help patients and their partners feel empowered, and take control of their pain. These techniques work- in fact they work *really well*. Unfortunately, once people stopped doing them, the pain would sometimes return- and I had to then hear patients say "my pain came back." I've heard from reliable sources that the same thing often happens in other physician's offices; the treatment helps patients find relief, but once the treatment ends, the pain can creep back. Sometimes it can be days or weeks, other times months or years- but nevertheless, more often than anyone would like, it returns. I remain convinced that we weren't designed to walk around in pain, and I have no desire to see everyone strung out on aspirin (or worse!). What was the missing step from the process? What was the elusive element that would make the difference between a temporary respite, and long- term relief?

That friends, is the sixty-four thousand dollar question. You want to know what that element is? I'm assuming you do, after all you *did* buy the book. So, right here, at the beginning of this book, let me give you a spoiler. The elusive end-all, be-all, cure-all for your back pain is this: The missing step, the elusive element, that one thing you need to address- is *everything*.

What?!?! *Everything? Are you freaking serious? REALLY?!?! I spent my hard- earned cash on Dr. Kirschner's book for him to tell me the path to relief is EVERYTHING?!?!* That sounds just a bit overwhelming, doesn't it? Everything. You're probably asking yourself 'What the hell does he mean by that?!?! You mean *everything* is causing my pain?' Well, yes. Observations I've made with patients, friends, and family have led me to really think about what makes someone's pain return after we've gone to Herculean efforts to make it go away, and the culprit is often a ginormous list of problems. Most people completely ignore these problems, setting them up for failure and a subsequent return to their doctor's office. Let me explain.

With the exception of a traumatic injury, back pain is almost always the cumulative effect of a host of factors (many of which we are going to go over in just a few short pages). When you treat the pain, but do little to eliminate all of those contributing factors that brought it about in the first place, you're probably going to be back in my office dealing with back pain again- frustrated, uncomfortable, and handing over yet *another* co-pay.

In this book, we will begin to examine many of those lifestyle factors, and give you simple, safe, and *effective* ways to fix them.

We will identify and then take steps to diffuse your *'anatomic bombs'*- the term I've come up with for the lifestyle and ergonomic traps we all have lurking around us. Simply eliminating these gremlins can go a long way towards getting the pain out of your life *forever*. The trick, however, is to first identify these problem areas, and then have the knowledge and expertise to *fix* them. This book will walk you through different aspects of your day-to-day life, and give you a series of things you can easily do to remove the obstacles between you and feeling *great!*

As you look through some of these suggestions, you'll likely say to yourself 'Well, that's obvious! Thanks for the tip, Einstein.' While that may be the case, I can state this with reasonable certainty: You are complicit with some of those supposedly obvious instances of self-sabotage. Furthermore, even though many of these tips may seem small, the cumulative effects of these simple lifestyle changes can be huge. Give them a shot. Even if you think they don't apply to you. Even if you think they are silly and won't make any difference. Even if you are totally convinced your back pain will never go away *no matter what you do*- give them a shot. You *did* things to cause your back pain- likely even things you were totally unaware were contributing to your pain when you did them. If you are reading this, you've already figured out that your pain isn't going to go away on its own. You are going to have to *do* things to rid yourself of it.

A lot can happen in six years...

There's one last thing I want to touch upon before we get into the thick of it. Let me share the first of several cautionary tales. The very same week I released my first book, *Back Together,* six years ago, my wife, Donna, gave birth to our second daughter. This exciting period of time seems like such a blur as I think about it now. The whole combination of events was completely overwhelming. While by and large my family was enjoying some wonderful things, there was just so much going on. Our new baby, Maya, had some complications associated with her birth, and spent several days in neonatal intensive care. Ultimately she was fine, but when we were able to finally bring her home, we had all of the new responsibility associated with a new baby including acclimating our older daughter, Ella, to her younger sibling. Those of you with children likely understand that this is no easy task. At the same time this was all happening, I was in full book-promotion mode, and was running all over the East Coast trying to get my message out: book signings, TV appearances, radio interviews. Most of the time it was fun and exciting, but it was well and truly exhausting all the same.

All of this excitement began to take a toll on both Donna and me. Little things started to happen. I was late on paying my cell phone bill. I missed a lunch meeting here or there. Donna would forget to call someone back. I started running chronically late during office hours. My wife would have a rough time with the kids in the morning and call me stressed out- looking for help which I just didn't know how to provide. As I think back in retrospect, I wasn't as supportive as I might have otherwise been, as I was pretty stressed out myself. Each one, in and of itself a relatively minor issue- but collectively they represented the smoldering embers of what would eventually turn into a wildfire. All of these little signs and symptoms continued to accumulate, until one fateful day several months later; I came home from the office and noticed something wasn't right- Donna wasn't herself. Her speech was broken and repetitive, and she had a difficult time even completing a sentence. I knew she was in trouble, and called a psychiatrist friend, who came straight over.

After a few minutes, it was clear that the situation had become serious, and I needed to get Donna some care right away. We went straight to the emergency department and there she was diagnosed with complications from severe postpartum depression. She was hospitalized for over a week, and when she came home we faced a long, slow recovery. It was nearly a year before I felt like I had my wonderful wife fully back in our lives.

A week or two after Donna returned home from the hospital, for the first time in my life, I woke up with back pain that I couldn't explain.

Up until that point, the only time I had ever experienced back pain was following a car accident, which occurred during my internship. The pain from that accident had resolved years before this incident. This pain was intense. It was something new and I didn't like it. I could have chalked my new back pain up to just about any number of things: I was stressed out of my gourd. My sleep was bad. I had gained about 15 pounds due to stress eating. I wasn't exercising. I wasn't paying attention to all of the ergonomic things I was telling my patients to do pretty much every day. How could I even begin to sift through all of these potential contributing factors? Which one caused my back to hurt? How's this sound for an answer- get ready for it- **ALL OF THEM!** (This is going to be a recurring theme in this book. Remember I told you the problem was *everything.)*

Earlier, when I told you the cause of your pain was all encompassing, this is what I meant. There were just *so many* contributing factors- it would have been impossible to point a finger at any one of them and say 'That's the one!' My pain was the result of potentially *dozens* of factors acting cumulatively, and all simultaneously exacerbated by my stress levels, which had me feeling like I was at DEFCON ONE for months on end.

Now, my personal example is extreme. Most people don't have the huge convergence of life changing events that we had (but you could) but we all have problems, issues and distractions going on in our lives. These distractions make it difficult to attend to important things such as fitness, or sleep, or daily ergonomics. I'm not berating anyone for this- it happens to *everyone*- including *me*, and including *you*. You may already be doing things to prevent back pain, perhaps even by accident. That's great. But let me tell you this; *your lifestyle is also contributing to your back pain.* I will show you how to use your lifestyle to get rid of it.

As you begin to go through the information in this book, I encourage you to do some groundwork so that you can get the most out of the suggestions I give you.

First and foremost, keep an open mind. As I said earlier, some of these suggestions may seem obvious at first, and you may tell yourself 'that couldn't possibly be a source of my pain.' Listen to what I am about to tell you, because this is key: ANYTHING and EVERYTHING can be a possible source of your pain. I may ask you to change some of your long-standing daily routines- and in some instances you may find these changes uncomfortable. Right off the bat, I'm going to ask you to try to be okay with them, and bear with me as we work to create your back-friendly lifestyle.

Second, I always subscribe to the notion that both success and failure leave clues. These clues may help you sort through problems and find simple solutions for your back pain. Starting *today,* begin to pay careful attention to the clues; here's a second use for that notebook- keep a back pain diary. Maintain a list of your daily activities, and keep a subjective rating of the severity of your pain on a scale from one to ten. As you collect some data over several weeks, you might notice patterns emerge. It may become clear that some activities make your pain worse, while others may help. These patterns may not immediately jump out at you, but the more you look, the more likely you will find information that points to possible sources of pain, and more importantly, sources of relief. In dealing with my patients, and with my own back pain, I can confidently state that this is one of the most useful diagnostic tools around- better than an x-ray, an MRI or anything else I could prescribe. Why? Because your pain diary serves as a snapshot of *your* life. It reveals the activities and other lifestyle factors that serve as *your* unique anatomic-bombs, and conversely, some of the defusing agents that help you to feel better.

Lastly, as you begin to construct your back-friendly lifestyle (which you must), and eliminate the anatomic bombs from your life and find some relief (and you will), decide here and now that you will stick with whichever changes you make that work the best. Going to the chiropractor, osteopath, massage therapist, physical therapist- or *anyone* for that matter who you may go to for relief can be a lot like drug addiction; we mentally acclimate ourselves to the idea that we need this treatment for relief, and it becomes a dependency.

Recovering addicts are given a set of psychological tools in rehab that help them to stay out of trouble, to remain clean, and to reduce their dependency on drugs or alcohol. Let this book guide you to discovering a primary set of tools for reducing your back pain. Simply having these tools will put you at an advantage over others who choose to just 'deal' with their pain. So many people walk around believing *nothing* they do will help their pain (except maybe popping some more pain killers), so they don't give too much thought to how their activities can really affect it. For example, if you've got chronic low back pain, you may already realize that carrying your two-year old kid around can make it worse. However, knowing this, did you ever experiment with any other types of child carriers, which may help you avoid the pain? How about this: does your pain only appear when you are sitting in your desk chair? Did you ever try another chair? Or how about moving things on your desk around in an effort to support your back? If you are like many people, you may have already identified a whole bunch of activities that make your pain worse, so you avoid them. But if you are like most people, you probably never really assembled a list of things that could *help* your pain (other than perhaps compiling a list of the things you *can't* do.) How great will it be to start making a list of all of the things you *can do* instead?

Everyone's back issues are unique. While sometimes you might need more aggressive tools such as osteopathic treatment, chiropractic adjustment, or even surgery to fix it, you owe it to yourself to optimize the various elements of your life to reduce the pain, and minimize it's effect on your life before necessarily resorting to those modalities. Let this book serve as the basic toolkit for recovering from back and neck pain, and for staying out of pain. Learn about these tools and use them. They will help you find your way to the pain-free lifestyle.

Use your best resource...

At the heart of my *Back Together* program is the notion that your loved one, be it a spouse, partner, child- even a friend, niece or nephew can serve as a valuable resource in helping you to recover from pain. In the program, I teach couples how to perform simple hands-on techniques with each other to help maintain normal function of the spine. The techniques are similar to those I use in my office, with much of the intimidating and potentially dangerous technical stuff taken out.

While I don't aim this book specifically at couples, you should certainly draw upon this valuable resource if you have a loved one available to work with as you go through this process. Let's face it: who has more at stake in you feeling well than your partner or spouse? Your pain probably affects them almost as much as it bothers you, and in my own experience in my medical practice, I've seen couples literally torn apart by the effects of chronic pain.

If you have a partner to work with:

Let them know that you are taking steps towards living a pain-free lifestyle. Simply letting them know your plan can be motivational -for *both of you*. You will feel a sense of commitment following your declaration, and hopefully, they will support your efforts.

Make a plan. After you have read through this book, create a list of the changes you plan to make *right now*. Go through the list with your partner, and see if they have additions they might suggest based upon their observations and knowledge of your individual situation.

Invite your partner to join you. Even if they have no pain, the ideas in this book can help you to *prevent* pain from cropping up in the future, so invite your partner to participate in any of the regular routines you choose to do -for example, your morning stretch. Much like a workout partner, doing this together can help keep you motivated and on track. As well, you'll both benefit from the ways that you modify your space in a back-friendly manner.

A few thoughts about pain...

Have you ever given much thought to why you have pain in the first place? It seems all of our bodily functions serve some purpose. Why then do we have pain? What is its purpose? The short answer is that pain is a self-preservation mechanism. It tells you there's something wrong, and that you had better do something about it (Take your hand away from the fire, turn down volume of the music, sit down and rest.) In more severe circumstances, pain can tell you to take more aggressive action (make an appointment to see your physician) or worse (call 911.)

Back pain tells you specific information about the position and condition of your spine. However, you need both willingness and the ability to listen to what it's saying- rather than telling yourself it will eventually go away, or worse- that you just have to live with it. Simply put, back pain is a warning system telling you one of two possible bits of information: 1) Some activity you are doing or have done recently is creating a mechanical condition which puts you at risk for damage, or 2) Some activity you've been doing for some time has caused damage, creating a mechanical condition which prevents normal function. Both factors result in even more pain. Keep these two bits of information in the back of your mind as you begin to think about your own back pain situation.

All-Pro NFL legend, Brian Dawkins wrote the introduction for *Back Together*. In the foreword, he had a great metaphor for back pain. He suggested that back pain was like a fire alarm, and that taking pain killers for your discomfort was like pouring water onto the alarm, silencing it, but letting the fire continue to burn down your house.

Have you been silencing the alarm without putting out the fire? If you've been hurting for a while, is it because you just didn't know what to do? Or, like so many people, were you simply convinced that there was really nothing you *could* do about your pain? Maybe you knew someone who threw their back out, and they were screwed up from that day on- so you figured if they couldn't fix their pain you wouldn't be able to do anything to fix yours either (I call this situation The Cousin Murray Pain Paradox or the TCMPP- Your cousin Murray threw his back out, and *he was never the same again*- so that became your understanding of just how back pain works.)

Let me make another very important point right here: **There are very few types of back pain that**

cannot be improved with care and attention. That said, it takes a good deal of courage to confront a problem like this, especially if your overall quality of life has been severely compromised by pain. You may have had multiple experiences informing your belief that pain was something you simply had to learn to live with. If you have been walking around in pain for a long time- hell- for any period of time, let me congratulate you on taking active steps towards giving your body the care and attention needed to finally make your pain go away. You have graduated from the ranks of people who either do nothing, or purchase books, videos & other programs only to have them languish in dust on the shelf, and up to the place where you have become an agent for your own well being. ***Back pain does not control you- you control your pain!***

I believe that the more information you have, the more you will understand why applying certain suggestions and tips will yield results. Then you will understand how to fine tune things to get even better results.

As you start to think about your own pain, and what you will do about it, you also need to recognize that there are several unique components to your pain- what I used to call the pain triad. Since my first book, I've realized I should have added another side to my model of pain. Unfortunately the result is a *pain trapezoid,* which honestly doesn't sound nearly as cool as a *triad*- but hey- sometimes you just gotta sacrifice form for function. Let's take a brief look at the four parts of my paradigm for pain- the newly christened "Pain Trapezoid":

The Pain Trapezoid

Physical   Lifestyle

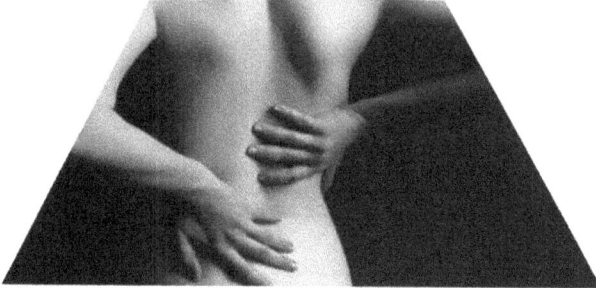

Neurological   Psychological

Physical: The first facet of the Pain Trapezoid is the physical cause of your pain. In most cases, some physical problem contributes to your pain- it could be something as simple as slight difference in the length of your legs, a muscle strain from lifting something too heavy, or something as severe as a broken bone. These physical problems can usually be identified in a physical examination or radiological study. They can be addressed by physical means (such as getting a small lift for your shoe, getting some physical therapy, or in the case of a broken spine- a body cast.) If you have a medical condition causing your pain, you will need to address this issue first. Without having a clear cause, or *diagnosis* of the primary cause of your pain, you won't be able to create an effective plan for ridding yourself of it. Before you go to the trouble of incorporating all of the thoughts I share with you in this book, be sure to consult your physician if you haven't already, and establish the *physical* cause of your pain. (In the next section, I shall give you a brief primer on the anatomy and physiology of pain so that you will better understand what your diagnosis actually means, and why some of the lifestyle modifications and suggestions I share with you will make a difference.)

At this point, one may ask, "why would I need to do anything else if I've fixed the problem?" Remember that part earlier where I said physicians hate to hear that someone's pain came back? Well, here is where that problem rears its seriously ugly head: You see, clinical experience has shown me that when dealing with back pain, treating the physical problem just doesn't do the trick. The pain goes away for a while, but then it comes back. Plenty of people walk around with slightly different length legs, irregularly shaped vertebrae, poor posture, bad discs, and a whole host of other potentially problematic physical findings. Interestingly, despite all of these problems, many of these same folks *do not have back pain*. These individuals may spend their entire life without back pain- but they are set up for it, and given the right, unfortunate combination of circumstances, boom- *pain*. These people have all manner of underlying conditions- virtual time bombs ticking away inside of them. However it may take the introduction of small ergonomic problems to tip the scale and cause these underlying conditions to become clinically relevant, and result in back pain. Which brings us to the next facet of the trapezoid...

Lifestyle: The primary focus of this book, your lifestyle is often the component of the Pain Trapezoid that pushes you 'over the edge' so to speak- pushes you from feeling _fine_ to feeling _terrible_. If you have physiological conditions, which set you up for back problems in the first place, sometimes the simplest, smallest aspects of one of your daily activities can be all it takes to stir up trouble. These become the _anatomic bombs_ I warned you about. Like a private investigator, you will need to pay careful attention to details, think about each of the aspects of your life, and try to identify the specific elements that cause your back pain or prevent it from going away. Lifestyle modifications can go a long way but you must also address...

Psychological: The psychological amplifier forms the third facet of the pain trapezoid. It's the part of your mind that modifies your perception of pain. When things in your life are going badly, or you are down or depressed, you will experience your pain in a very different way than if, for instance, you just learned you won the Powerball. You cannot underestimate the psychological contribution to your pain. Pay it the attention it deserves. I will give you some of my thoughts on how to better manage the psychological aspects of your pain in a little bit, but before we continue, I want to clarify something. If you expect me to tell you that emotional stress is the *cause* of your back pain, let me put that idea to rest *now*. I know that several physicians and authors out there have made a lot of money telling you that your pain is purely a function of your stress. My clinical experience tells me this: *Stress does not **cause** anything.* Stress takes whatever underlying physiological condition you have, be it high blood pressure, ulcers, and yes, back pain- and it makes it worse. Stress is not a *causal* agent, but an *exacerbating* factor. And the last side of the trapezoid...

Neurological: Perhaps the most poorly understood component of the equation is the neurological portion of the trapezoid. Most people know that nerves are the part of the body that *feel* pain, but they can also be the part of your body that makes you continue to suffer, even when things have otherwise healed up. This phenomenon is what I refer to as the Learned Neurological Response, or LNR. The best way I have found to describe the LNR is through the analogy of playing a musical instrument: When musicians first pick up a new piece of music to learn, they will practice the piece over and over- getting better each time. This repetition creates a series of neural pathways that they can access whenever they want to play the piece, and the more they repeat the piece, the more deeply entrenched these pathways become. The really interesting thing about this process is that if they put down the piece for a long time (perhaps months, or even years) and then play it again, they probably won't be able to play it perfectly, but they will perform the piece significantly better than when they first picked it up. This happens because once the player has established those pathways, they can be very hard to eliminate.

In the same way, when you are injured, or you have engaged in an activity with bad ergonomics or poor body mechanics, your body may have established an alternative or damaged series of pathways or *firing patterns* in an effort to find less painful ways of performing routine tasks. These damaged pathways are very difficult to unlearn, and come in two varieties: those patterns established for the purpose of finding less painful ways of doing activities which had become painful, and those pathways which are very efficient at feeling pain- because that's what they were created to do. Either of these can prolong your discomfort, and make it much more difficult to shake: being in pain forces your body to try to modify activities to make them less painful, reinforcing the already compromised situation.

You may have gone to a chiropractor, an osteopath, an internist- it doesn't really matter what type of practitioner you visited- and they may have treated your immediate physical ailment and made your pain go away- temporarily. However, if there were circumstances in your life that allowed these physical conditions to happen in the first place, which went unaddressed, your pain likely returned (and I already told you, I *hate* that- and it's pretty clear you do too- again having bought the book and everything.)

Anatomy 101...

If you've ever seen images of the spine in a textbook or online the whole thing can look pretty complicated. All of the names doctors use to describe the anatomical structures and the conditions that afflict them, make things sound even more intimidating. However, if you take the time to break things down into the basics, the spine is actually a pretty straightforward mechanism, and is relatively easy to understand.

There's a model I use when teaching medical students in my office that helps me explain how to diagnose the origin of a patient's pain. The paradigm I've developed breaks down the spine into its basic elements, and simplifies how I identify the specific physical structure that causes a patient pain. I hope this model will help you to understand the physical origins of your own pain.

At any level in your spine, from your neck all the way down to your tailbone, there are pretty much only five possible structures that are capable of causing you pain. Really. No matter your diagnosis, there are only these five possible things, which repeat thirty times from the top down to the bottom of your spine. There are a couple of exceptions (specifically fractures and cancer), but by and large these five things are generally the culprits:

Vertebrae, the bones of your spine, have several parts. For our purposes here, the most important parts are what are known as the *facets,* or the joints that articulate your spine. The shape of the facets dictates what kind of movements their associated vertebrae can make. For example, the facets in the neck allow lots of types of movement; side to side, rotation left or right, and looking up and down, allowing you to turn your head efficiently to be able to pay attention to your surroundings. Conversely, the facets in the lumbar spine are not particularly good at rotation or sidebending, but do a great job with flexion and extension, allowing you to efficiently sit or stand, and to lift heavy objects. Like any of your moveable joints, they are susceptible to osteoarthritis and inflammation due to overuse.

Intervertebral discs are frequently blamed (too often in fact) for a disproportionate amount of back pain (your cousin Murray probably has a herniated disc!) Discs are the shock absorbers between your vertebrae. They prevent the jarring forces of most weight-bearing activity from being transmitted up to your head. Without them, activities as benign as _walking_ would cause you a concussion. Intervertebral discs also hold the vertebrae together. The disc is made out of two primary structures; the _nucleus pulposa,_ which is the soft inner core of the disc, and the _annulus fibrosa,_ which is the thick, fibrous ring around the disc which holds everything in. Discs are susceptible to degeneration due to wear and tear, but most commonly people worry about a bulging or *herniated* disc. A herniation occurs when the annulus is weakened or damaged and pressure inside the disc causes it to bulge outward and potentially impinge upon the movement of a joint surface or worse, put pressure on a nerve. For example, some cases of sciatic pain are caused when a disc bulges out and presses on the nerve that emerges between the lowest lumbar vertebra and the first sacral vertebra.

Nerves perform two primary functions. First, they send instructions out to the rest of the body, directing various actions- for example, sitting, standing, reading, or bending. Second, they transmit signals from the body back to your brain. These signals can contain information about position, danger- such as extreme heat, or telling you- in the case of back pain- that something is wrong. Nerves can cause pain when they are impinged, or when there is some other mechanical problem. Also, they can be a secondary source of pain when you have disrupted firing patterns resulting in disrupted or inappropriate body mechanics. For example, if someone has had an accident or fall, they may have begun to favor one side of their body over the other in an effort to avoid pain. Their traumatic injuries could completely resolve, but their body can become acclimated to the modified way of doing things (remember those pathways established by the LNR?), so they continue to favor the previously less painful side. Over time this can result in wear and tear due to areas being placed under new stress.

Muscles can only do two things: contract or relax. When they contract, they cause movement of some part of the body. When they relax, they allow the body part to return to its previous position. Almost all muscles have an opposing muscle that does the opposite action- for example, your biceps muscle flexes your arm (bends it), and your triceps muscle extends it (straightens it out.) Muscles can be strained when overworked with too much activity, or torn when they are overburdened with too much weight or resistance. Strains and sprains typically heal well with rest, as do minor tears. More serious tears occasionally require surgical intervention to reconnect the separated ends of the muscle. Strains and tears can be painful conditions depending upon the severity.

Everything else. Here I group all of the structures that hold everything together, including ligaments, tendons, and connective tissue. These structures interact with just about every moving structure in your body: Tendons connect muscle to bone. Ligaments connect bone to bone. Broad sheets of connective tissue bind everything together, and allow for the passage of cellular waste products gathered by the lymphatic system. As with muscles, tendons and ligaments can be strained or sprained. However, due to a less active blood supply, these structures typically take a good deal longer to heal when injured. Connective tissue can develop trigger points and tender points. It is theorized that these painful points occur when cellular waste aggregates between layers of connective tissue, and have a difficult time being cleared.

So, in spite of the enormous variety of conditions, and the apparent complexity of the anatomy involved, these five structures are the culprits in an overwhelming variety of painful neck and back conditions. Problems with any of them can cause instability or additional problems with the others. As you consider some of the lifestyle modifications you plan to pursue, try to think about how these five structures might be involved. Also note that, in many cases, painful conditions may involve more than one structure, and the more you pay attention, the more you'll be able to understand how they intermingle and affect each other.

Here's an extreme example: A man falls and bruises his left hip. He then favors the right hip, as the left is more painful. Because of the added load, the right sacroiliac joint becomes dysfunctional (stops moving appropriately). The *Piriformis* muscle, which stabilizes the sacrum becomes spasmic in response to the dysfunctional joint, and because of the spasm, thickens in the middle. Because the Piriformis is enlarged in its center, it presses down on the sciatic nerve, resulting in sciatic pain in the right leg, which then causes the person to favor the *left* leg. Can you see how the whole cycle perpetuates itself? A physician might treat any one of the conditions in that dynamic chain, and still not resolve their patient's pain. I don't expect you to necessarily follow all of the 'dominos' which may be causing *your* pain- hopefully your doctor or therapist will help you with that. What I would like you to do is to start thinking about how any one of these lifestyle modifications might affect one or more of the five structures we just reviewed. Switching to this way of thinking will not only help you to fix the pain you have now, but will also help you to recognize potential anatomic bombs *before* they have a chance to cause you pain!

As you read this book and begin to think about how to utilize the suggestions you find, try to keep the elements of the trapezoid in the back of your mind. Are you paying attention to all four? *(Hint: You should consider including this in your journal.)*

Where to start?

As you read this book, and after you are finished- make the commitment to honestly take a few minutes out of each and every day to really think about which suggestions you've adopted, and which you would like to take advantage of right now and then *do* them. Do them. DO THEM!! Together, we shall create a back-friendly lifestyle. And like any lifestyle modification process, you really need to think about the process and take action *every single day* in order for it to be effective. This is not a New Years resolution which you can forget about a few weeks from now and still expect results. This requires a commitment to a back-friendly life, a change in your lifestyle that will provide you benefits *forever*. Thousands of people have done the things in this book and achieved results. And with some real dedication, you will too! I've already given you one way to help you keep this commitment: maintaining a pain journal. But let me give you two additional assignments to help keep you on track:

-Commit to applying one or two of the suggestions you read here in the book every couple of days. Slowly accumulate a list of things you have changed to make your lifestyle more back-friendly. A longer-lasting ability to keep up with these changes will come with their gradual application, rather than jumping in and trying to change everything all at once. It is like the difference between a crash diet and a long-term nutrition plan: One may help you lose weight for a short while but the weight will likely come back; the other will give you long-term changes. At the beginning of each day, before you even get out of bed, decide what you will do for your back that day. At the end of the day, ask yourself what things you did to support your back that day- and if you can say you did something- no matter how small it might be- you are on your way.

-One of the tools I use in my office to help keep track of a patients progress is the Subjective Pain Analysis, or SPA. The SPA divides your body into different regions, and allows you to subjectively rate on a scale from 0-10, how much pain you are experiencing in each of those regions. In your journal, you should be rating your overall, general level of discomfort on a scale of one to 10. In the SPA, you will be more specific with each area of your body. Fill out an SPA once every couple of weeks and keep track of how you are doing. There's a copyable SPA in the back of this book. A printable version can be downloaded from my websites, www.backtogether.org and www.backtogethercentral.com. As you chart your progress, some of the changes you experience will be subtle. Charting them so you have visual evidence of your progress can really motivate you -like getting on the scale when you are dieting and discovering that you've lost a few pounds.

Part II: The Walk

As a physician, I generally address a patient's physical problems first- coming up with a clear diagnosis for their discomfort and then treating it. This treatment can come in the form of prescription medications, manual medicine, physical therapy or others. However, when I first interview a new patient, I will also ask a whole host of questions about their pain in order to help me get to the where, when, how, and why of the pain. I learn about their work, their sleep habits, their home life, hobbies, their medical history, their parents' medical history and a lot more. This information is one of the starting points from which I create a long-term treatment plan for that patient. This book will address many of the questions I ask in my initial interview. As you read each section, you may immediately know that a certain suggestion does not apply to your situation (*most* men don't have to deal with high heels.) If you are even a little unsure if something applies to you, try it anyway. There is nothing in this book that will hurt you, and you may be surprised how much some tips help you. Remember, *small things can have enormous effects.*

Your home.

Your home is as good a place to start as any for a whole bunch of reasons, not the least of which are 1) you probably spend more time there than anywhere else and 2) it is likely the place where you have the most control over your environment, so you have the greatest opportunity to effect positive change.

Before we get into some of the specific rooms in your home, take a few minutes to walk around and check things out. Notice how your furniture is positioned, where you keep the household items you commonly use, as well as which parts of your home you occupy most often. The Eastern concept of *Feng Shui* has become quite popular of late and it is interesting to note that many of the suggestions found in a complete Feng Shui assessment of a home will also result in a home that is more back-friendly. If you pay careful attention as you tour through your home, you may actually recognize some of the anatomic bombs there before you even read my thoughts on how to set things right. As I forewarned you, while we investigate the various parts of your life- starting with your home, I may ask you to change some things here and there- some things which you may have had your certain way since you were a child- so try not to be too wedded to your current conditions.

Your bedroom

The morning can be a really tough time for many people with back pain. An overwhelming number of people tell me that the morning is the worst time of the day for them. Additionally, the morning seems to be the time of day most patients 'throw their backs out.' Several reasons lurk behind this phenomenon:

1) When you arise, your joints and muscles have not had a chance to warm up, resulting in stiffness. This stiffness can change your body mechanics sufficiently to actually set you up for injury, as your body subconsciously tries to find less painful ways of doing things. Consequently, people with osteoarthritis (who tend to be the stiffest in the morning) are particularly susceptible to problems during this time of day.

2) Everyone's sleep habits differ and these variations can make it tough to adjust when you first get out of bed. For example, I generally try to talk patients out of sleeping on their abdomens. This sleep position leaves the lumbar *and* cervical spine in an extended position for prolonged periods. This puts strain on the intervertebral discs exactly in the spots where they are most vulnerable. The problems caused by these unpredictable, often physiologically stressful sleep positions are often further exacerbated by the fact that...

3) Many people stay in bed until the last possible moment, trying to eke out those last seconds of rest before starting their days. Consequently, many folks find themselves rushing out of bed and spinning around their bedrooms like the Tasmanian Devil trying to get to work on time- really not the optimal way to begin the day.

Of course, these are just a few of the contributing factors...

There are some things you can (*must!*) do, to make your morning less risky, and they all start with a good night's sleep.

One of the key things I tell patients over and over is that they must *defend their sleep* above almost anything else. Sleep is time to recover from your daily activity: time for your brain to clear and time for your body to recharge, recover, and reset. For many, sleep is the only time that is truly *theirs*- a time when they are not beholden to any other responsibilities. Quality sleep can help make waking up a lot less painful, and lessen the likelihood that you will further harm yourself. Conversely, *nothing* can botch your day more than being poorly rested.

Despite the clear necessity for quality sleep, I find it astonishing how poorly some patients treat themselves with regard to this important aspect of self-maintenance. What's also remarkable to me is what a difference this one thing has on an individual's pain. If you change *nothing* else, giving yourself quality rest will make it less likely that you will further injure yourself, reduce the effects of back and neck pain on your daily life, and generally make your life more comfortable. There are some relatively simple things you can do to help improve the quality of your sleep right away. If your pain actually interrupts your sleep, following these tips may help you reduce your discomfort, and hopefully break this destructive cycle:

First things first- you've got to make sure your bedroom is a welcoming place for rest. Physicians refer to this as *sleep hygiene,* (warm & fuzzy, no?) Try these suggestions to help improve the quality of your sleep:

Darken your bedroom. Even with your eyes closed, your body responds to ambient light. A thin portion of bone behind your eyes allows small amounts of light to penetrate through to the inside of your head. This small amount of light can be sensed by a tiny organ known as the *pineal gland*, which is partially responsible for the regulation of your sleep cycle. Even dim light can send your body the message that it's morning and time to get up. You need to find a way to keep the room dark until you are ready to wake up. Streetlights and other ambient sources of light can undermine your sleep. If closed blinds don't do the job, blackout curtains can help. An eye mask or even a dark colored sheet hung over the window frame are inexpensive alternatives.

A quiet bedroom is key. If you live in a high

traffic area, or, worse, you sleep with someone who snores, you already understand what an impact noise can have on your sleep. I have too much anxiety to sleep with ear plugs as I'm always afraid I will miss something (you know- like say, a fire alarm), but many people find them to be a good solution for blocking unwanted sounds while sleeping. A white noise generator is a great way to reduce the effects of ambient noise. You can find literally hundreds of cost-effective solutions available from myriad sources, both in retail shops and on the Internet.

Don't sleep on an ancient bed. During my intake interview with any new back pain patient, I always ask about the age of their mattress. I find it bewildering how many people don't even remember when they got their mattress. Here's a loose rule: If you don't remember when you got your mattress, it's probably time to get a new one (also a great guideline for when to get a tetanus shot.) Old mattresses will eventually lose their resiliency, and sag in the center where the majority of your body weight lays. This makes it impossible for the mattress to do its primary job- supporting your body in a comfortable, neutral position. People frequently ask me what kind of mattress I recommend but I usually shy away from this question. Everyone's sleep habits differ (you wouldn't believe how much flack I get from my friends because Donna and I sleep on a hard, traditional Japanese tatami mat. It's great for us- but you'd probably hate it) so it's hard to make a, ahem, *blanket* recommendation. I generally suggest that you go with a firm supportive mattress, and if possible purchase from a company that has a liberal exchange policy- some stores will let you try out a mattress (in a mattress cover of course) and exchange it if you find it isn't doing the trick. If you have back pain, avoid waterbeds like the plague- in fact, even if you don't have back pain, they are a pretty bad idea, as they simply cannot support the weight of your midsection. Use supportive pillows, which allow you to maintain as neutral a position for your neck as possible (not extended all the way up if you sleep on your back, and not side bent right or left if you sleep on your side.)

Appropriate bedding is a must. If you don't already, keep two types of sets of bedding- one for cold weather, and another for warm. I'm amazed how many people use the same comforter throughout the year. You don't need to spend a lot of money to have temperature appropriate bedding. The bottom line is that if you are comfortable, you're going to sleep better.

Quality sleep doesn't only have to do with what happens at nighttime- it also relates to what happens when you wake up.

Your Wake up call...

Like many, I am just not a morning person. I really like to take my time getting out of bed. I love lounging in bed with my wife. On weekends, I enjoy it when my kids come in and join us while we take a few minutes to talk about the things we want to do that day. In short, I really take my good, sweet time dragging my ass out of bed. It can be a really nice part of the day if you make the time, but it is also the time of day for you to take some of your first preventive measures to keep yourself pain-free:

If possible, get an alarm clock that does not annoy you. Sure, a loudly honking horn will get you out of bed, but being suddenly jarred out of a restful sleep is not a helpful way to begin a pain-free day. Being startled stimulates your adrenal glands and can activate the sympathetic part of your central nervous system. This can cause your muscles to get even tighter. If you cannot find an alarm clock with a pleasant wake-up sound, try a clock radio tuned to a station you like, or better yet, a clock with an option to play a CD or iPod loaded with music you know you like. In keeping with improving the psychological component of *your* pain trapezoid, taking steps to not wake up abruptly or with annoying sounds (such as any music in the Top 40 after, say, 1987), will set you off on the right foot for the rest of your day.

Set your wake-up alarm a few minutes earlier than you think you will need it.

This serves several purposes. First, it will give you time to start your day gradually, rather than rushing. Second, it will give you an opportunity to...

Take a few minutes to gently stretch out your muscles and move joints that may have stiffened during sleep. As I related earlier, the morning is one of the most common times to 'throw out your back.' This often happens while people do something as unremarkable as putting on their socks. A gentle stretch will reduce your risk of injury by restoring any range of motion lost to stiffness that occurred during sleep. It will also reduce some of the effects of pain you may already have. A gentle stretch will also help get your body ready for the rest of the day. You really only need three or four minutes to mobilize your body. Try this simple sequence:

1) Extend your whole foot towards the base of your bed,pointing your toes straight down, and hold for about 5-10 seconds.

2) Flex your foot up towards your head, stretching out

the backs of your calves and heels, and hold for about 5-10 seconds.

3) Bend your knees, and, with your feet and hips on the bed, allow your knees to gently lower towards one side and then the other, allowing the outer knee to rest on the bed. Hold each side for about 5-10 seconds.

4) Bring each knee individually up to your chest, and hold there for about 5-10 seconds on each side.

5) Bring both knees simultaneously up to your chest, and hold for about 5-10 seconds.

6) From a laying position, extend both of your arms straight up towards the ceiling, and hold for about 5-10 seconds.

7) Turn your head both to the right and to the left as far as you can comfortably rotate, and hold each direction for about 5-10 seconds.

8) Sit up in your bed with your legs hanging over the side of the bed, and reach your arms over your head

towards the ceiling, holding for about 5-10 seconds.

9) Slowly stand on your feet. As you stand, again reach your arms up towards the ceiling, inhaling deeply as you reach up towards the ceiling, again holding for about 5-10 seconds.

10) Take three slow, deep cleansing breaths (I'll discuss some of the significant benefits of deep breathing exercises shortly.)

11) Reach over and pat yourself on the back- you probably have just woken up correctly for the first time since you were an infant!

Sleep and wake-up time are the foundation of your day. In much the same way that you would build a strong foundation for your home or a building, give your day the strong foundation it needs. These steps will get you out of bed and out the door with less pain, less risk of injuring yourself, and better equipped to deal with your day.

And since we are already in the bedroom...

There's this pained look patients get on their face right before they ask me about sex and back pain- and it is the same look whether they are men or women, whether they are young or old, and no matter where they are from.

Unfortunately, when people are in pain, sexual intimacy is one of the first activities that often gets pushed aside. In addition to concerns about the potential physical discomfort that *might* occur, there are psychological reasons for this as well; back pain can make people feel diminished and damaged. Anxiety about potentially disappointing sexual performance due to pain can add to these feelings. The irony is that while people often stop engaging in sexual activity when they are in pain, more often than not, sex will actually help *reduce* their discomfort. The slow, gentle pulsing of sexual activity can help to mobilize segments in the spine that have become, for lack of a better term, stuck. An orgasm stimulates the release of endorphins, which have a natural pain-reducing effect. Furthermore, when a couple that has lost closeness due to ongoing pain can restore their intimacy, they can bring back a sense of normalcy for both partners. This can enhance and bolster the psychological corner of the pain trapezoid.

Here's the problem: Many people recovering from various types of back pain initially find sex uncomfortable; it can actually exacerbate their pain. This typically happens when individuals have a fixed definition of what constitutes sexual intimacy. This is definitely an area in which experimentation and innovation can reap huge rewards. You may find that as a couple, you may have to temporarily (and sometimes permanently) change your model of sexual activity. Trying different positions and play surfaces can often help to identify more comfortable variations; in extreme cases you may need to refrain from the traditional model of intercourse and try manual or oral stimulation, even perhaps enhancing your mutual pleasure with *aural* stimulation to get your other senses involved in the experience.

Whatever you do, don't give up: *sex is fun,* as well as physically and emotionally good for you. Something out there works for everybody. It may take some trial and error, but the rewards for all of your efforts and research will be huge for you *and* your partner.

The skeletons in your closet...

Every morning, whether on a workday or a weekend, you will deal with the contents of your closet. Your closet is probably an accomplice in perpetuating your back pain. All kinds of products and systems can help you to organize and arrange your closet. While most will help it to look neat, few if *any* focus on making your closet back-friendly. As before, let me remind you that some of my suggestions will sound small or perhaps less relevant. I also remind you that most back pain arises from a whole plethora of cumulative junk- so it may take a plethora of small, cumulative improvements to get yourself out of pain and feeling *great!*

Here are some tips for eliminating the anatomic bombs in your closet:

82

Set up a 'seasonal' closet. Only leave those clothing items you will need to access for that given season. Do you really need to be sorting through sundresses in December or sweaters in July? Put the other items in another closet, in storage boxes under your bed, or in your attic if you have one, replacing them when appropriate. This suggestion will help to simplify the next recommendation...

Unstuff your hanging garments. Even I am guilty of this one: having your closets' hanging racks so packed with shirts, etc., that you need to push hard against the contents just to get to the shirts/pants/dress you want to remove. Even in larger closets, this can force you to twist your lumbar spine while pushing things out of the way at the time of day when your body is least ready to deal with additional stressors. Thin out the herd: get rid of clothing you have not worn for a while (swap, sell, or donate!) Put less frequently used items into storage until you think you may wear them again.

Get your shoes off the floor!!! So many people keep their shoes on the floor of their closet, either in boxes, or even loose underneath their hanging garments. This is just asking for trouble, as you are forced to go into a position of extreme flexion and twisting just to pick out footwear. For under 10 dollars, you can purchase a shoe hanger that goes over the back of the closet door. This elevates your shoes closer to eye level, and reduces your risk of hurting your back.

Move the more accessed items, such as underwear and socks, up to a higher drawer to avoid going into extreme flexion reaching for things first thing in the day. I was having dinner with some friends while doing research for this book and on a lark, asked them in which drawer they keep their underwear and socks (Yeah, I got a few odd looks.) Interestingly, about two thirds of the dozen or so people present related that they kept them in the bottom drawers. Presumably, you wear underwear and socks most days. Move them to the top!

Lastly, try selecting your outfits for the next day the evening before. As I mentioned, your spine has had little time to warm up when you first climb out of bed in the morning. If you pull out all of the items you will need from your closet the night before and lay them out for easy access, you will both reduce the risk to your back, and feel less rushed as you get ready for your day.

And, since we are going through your closet anyway: Your Clothing

Last year I did a blog post on thebacktogetherblog.com discussing bras, and how an incorrectly sized bra can cause all sorts of havoc on a woman's spine. This particular post went viral and got picked up by a bunch of other blogs, health sites, and even Glamour Magazine. All of a sudden I was a lingerie guru as well- which, in all honesty, was kind of fun. While answering all sorts of questions from readers and patients about women's underwear, I began to really think about all of the other ways clothing can create anatomic bombs. Let's take a moment to go through some clothing issues that may be causing you trouble...

Trousers: Many men have a significant amount of their egos tied up in their pants size. They often cling to the same size pants they wore when they were younger, when they felt like they were at their physical peak, or as when they met their mate. Sadly, this is not always because they have remained the same size, but more because they have adjusted where their pants sit on their bodies. Often they drop their pants way too low under their gut *(see: Philadelphia- my home town)*, or hiked all the way up to their nipples *(see: Boca Raton.)*

Your waist size should be measured annually, or more frequently if you are involved in any sort of weight management program. You should keep your pants purchases correctly and *honestly* sized. Incorrectly sized pants can inadvertently restrict movement of the sacrum- and in particular, the sacroiliac joints- where the sacrum and the pelvic bones join. Additionally, the wrong sized pants can disrupt normal breathing mechanics by restricting movement of the diaphragm, and impede flexion & extension of the lumbar spine, which can cause all manner of troubles. Wear the correct size pants. Ok?

Jackets: Like pants, jackets should be correctly sized, and again, checked annually. Jackets should button or zip with a little extra room and be unrestrictive. To test the fit, pull your arms across to the opposite shoulders and note whether the jacket feels uncomfortably tight or restrictive. If it does, move up to the next size. When possible, stick with lighter weight jackets, and try not to weigh down your jacket with tons of stuff in the pockets. I see this particular problem occur most often with each new intern class in the hospitals in which I work: their newly pressed white lab coats weighed down with a hundred reference books, and all sorts of diagnostic paraphernalia. When combined with the stress of being a newly minted intern, it's no wonder most young doctors are walking around in pain! These heavily weighted coats put pressure on the first ribs (which are the skeletal *fulcrum* of your breathing mechanism) as well as the back of your neck, which can cause an exaggeration of the normal curvature of your cervical and thoracic spine. Wear the right sized coat and empty out your pockets!

Shirts: Wearing a shirt with the wrong sized collar can result in both neck pain (by restricting neck movement), and headaches (by limiting movement and placing compression on your carotid arteries). Be sure you can comfortably insert 3 fingers between your shirt and your neck. If you are wearing a tie, the same rule applies.

Bras: An informal study in my office in 2002 found that over fifty percent of women were wearing an incorrectly sized bra, and from that group, over seventy percent of the women examined had dysfunctional spinal segments at or near the level where their bra crossed over their backs. A bra which is too tight may *feel* as thought it is providing more support, but, in fact it may limit the normal inhalation and exhalation movements of the ribs and disrupt the normal mechanics of the thoracic spine.

I strongly recommend a routine bra fitting. While many better stores will offer the service, I discovered that some women are uncomfortable with it. Be personally uncomfortable for a few minutes- it is far better than being physically uncomfortable all the time. This one adjustment can take stress off of the upper back, significantly improve thoracic function, and diminish mid-back pain.

Underpants: As always, wear clean underpants. It won't help your back, but it just seems like a good idea.

Shoes: I could probably write an entire book on how shoes can affect back pain. They can play such a huge role in the health of your spine- particularly if you are wearing the _wrong_ shoes. As the foundation supporting all of your body weight, and the only external support your skeleton routinely gets, it is no surprise that shoes can play a serious role in how your back feels. There are many considerations; here are a few of my main points:

-Wear shoes with good arch support and cushioning when possible. Your arches are the first location of shock absorption for your musculoskeletal system. They decrease the amounts of shock transmitted throughout your entire body, even by such simple activities as walking. Unfortunately, most dress shoes provide little or no support. I realize that I have pretty much zero chance of convincing you to not wear them at all. Hopefully, you don't need to wear them that often. When possible, try to shop for shoes that provide a reasonable compromise between style and comfort/support. I know you want to look good- but having gorgeous designer shoes on your feet is easily overshadowed by walking around all hunched over with your face contorted in pain, looking for a comfortable place to sit down. Choose shoes with good arch support, some cushioning, and a flexible, shock-absorbing sole.

-Watch out for shoes that squish your toes together. Your toes are the launching pad for every step you take, and compressing them together will compromise your foot mechanics. This can then cause a cascade of mechanical consequences throughout your body.

-When you buy athletic shoes, stick with shoes designed for the activities you will actually perform. When I was a kid, you got 'sneakers.' These were general-purpose athletic shoes- and you used them for pretty much *everything*. Over the years, as shoe designers began to really understand the mechanics of various sporting activities, they started to change the shoe designs to accommodate different types of movement. Shoe manufacturers have given a tremendous amount of thought and research into the designs of athletic shoes, changing the shapes of the soles, the materials used, and the locations of the arch support to accommodate specific activities. We should all take advantage of their knowledge base. Running shoes appropriate for running. Walking shoes for walking. Tiddlywinks shoes appropriate for tiddlywinks. (I'm still waiting for someone to tell me what the hell tiddlywinks actually *is*.) Wear the appropriate shoes!

-The materials of all shoes will eventually lose their resiliency and compressibility; so do not hold onto *any* shoes for too long. This is particularly true for athletic shoes. The shoes you use to run on the indoor treadmill may *look* brand new, having never been exposed to the elements, but inside where it counts, they're not. Without the support and shock absorption offered by a pair of quality shoes, your arches will go unprotected. This can become a serious problem during higher impact activities. Worn out shoes can actually alter your foot mechanics as well. This plus the added stress of impact will put your spine at risk. Replace your shoes regularly. Oh, and as an aside, here's a valuable gem- if you find a pair of athletic shoes you *really* like, and that work particularly well for you- buy a few pairs the next time they go on sale. The right shoes can be like magic, and manufacturers change their lines often enough that you may find yourself unable to get the 'perfect shoe' for too long. On that note, if you happen to come across a few new-old-stock pairs of Avia 500's in size 11- PLEASE shoot me an email (For those of you who've been around a while, you know these are seriously old-school, but I wish I'd bought ALL of them.)

-When selecting high heels, try to stick with shoes that have a broad heel at the base, which will help to provide lateral support for your ankles, and help keep your back out of trouble. As I've said many times, mules are your friend. I own about 8 pairs of cowboy boots, all of which have approximately a one-inch heel. People are always surprised to hear me say that these are the most comfortable shoes I own- but they provide a tiny degree of pelvic tilt, have solid arch support, and have that broad heel I'm talking about.

-As is the case with any other pieces of clothing, correct sizing matters- in this case, probably even more so. Also note that shoe sizes can change with age and weight. Check periodically to be sure you've gotten the right size.

Belts: Belts should follow the same basic rules as pants: not too tight, not sitting on the sacrum, and in spite of any current or coming fashion trends, not too wide (not for any health reasons in particularly, but more so because they are simply ugly. Really.) Poorly sized belts can lock the sacrum and/or lumbar vertebrae into a fixed position, forcing the adjacent vertebrae to compensate for the lack of movement- and passing stress on up the spine.

Handbags or Briefcases: Once a week or so, take a few moments to empty the unnecessary contents of your briefcase or handbag. I can't believe how much junk I can accumulate in a week, and I know I am not alone with this problem: My mom has been known to carry a purse the size of a body bag, and I don't think she even remembers most of the stuff she's got in it- I'm pretty sure I once saw her pull a car battery out of her handbag.

Dump the contents of your bag onto a table or counter, and see what you really need, leaving behind the rest. Carrying the extra weight- particularly on one side or the other (most of us favor one)- puts your spine at risk for problems. If you can, try to periodically switch the side on which you carry your handbag or briefcase.

Where are we?

So now you're awake after a good night's sleep. You've gotten out of bed in a manner befitting someone looking to be out of pain. Perhaps if you're *really* lucky, you've had some great sex. You've gotten dressed with items carefully selected from a closet specifically designed to prevent back problems. Presumably, you've eaten a healthy and nutritious breakfast (I won't get into nutrition- that'll be the next book. In keeping with the overall theme of this book, be good to yourself and fuel up with good food. Chocolate Sugar Mega Crunch with marshmallow cartoon characters will not help your body to heal up. As in all things, remember to proceed with moderation and balance- treat your body well, and it will treat you well in return.) Once you've enacted some of these recommendations, you'll have taken the first steps towards defusing the morning anatomic bombs, and be well on your way towards living the pain-free lifestyle.

Alternatively, at this point you may have looked at this first group of suggestions and said to yourself "these are such small things- *there's just no way this is going to help my back pain.*" Well, let me give you two examples that help illustrate that there is nothing that is so small that it cannot make a difference, and hopefully make another point, which you may find valuable...

Small things...

A favorite anecdote I use to illustrate the concept of small things and their enormous effects comes from a car auction I attended with my dad when I was a kid, and involves a very rare Ferrari automobile (I am a serious car guy, and at that age being near that car was like standing next to a supermodel.) The car fetched a record price at auction but upon being started up, the engine sputtered and stalled- not the delightful sound we had all hoped to hear emitting from this fine and beautiful Italian sports car. Everyone just assumed that the engine was fried, but it took the knowledge of a little old man who once worked tuning Ferrari engines and a coin to set things right. With just the simple turn of a screw, using a dime as a screwdriver to adjust a carburetor, this man was able to solve the problem, and leave the car running perfectly.

This anecdote is a real-life variation of a story (which may or may not be urban legend- these things get passed around so much you can never really be sure,) involving a broken conveyor system at Federal Express. It seems that there was a package conveyor system at a FedEx hub somewhere that had broken down. The local director brought in a repair expert who went in, looked at the system for two minutes, took out a screwdriver, turned a screw a couple of turns, flipped a switch, and the whole system roared back to life. He then handed them a bill for five grand, which the supervisor refused to pay, demanding a detailed invoice of the costs involved in this two-minute repair for him to provide to *his* supervisor. The story ends with the repairman handing the supervisor an invoice that read "Adjusting the mechanism- $30, Knowing which screw to turn- $4970."

Ok, so that one's probably made up (in the corporate world, the supervisor probably didn't even look at the bill, faxed it to their accounting department, located three thousand miles away, and completely oblivious to the apparent absurdity of the bill in question, paid it anyway!), but both of these stories carry two very important messages:

First, to reiterate, *little things can have enormous effects;* some of the ideas presented in this book will seem minuscule, but their effects can often prove miraculous. If you need further convincing that these tiny things can make a difference, try this little experiment: pick a day, and move your wristwatch to your other hand. Why? You'll be absolutely shocked how much this one change can screw up your day. You will probably bang your watch into pretty much every doorframe you walk through. You'll look at the wrong wrist to check the time about a hundred times through your day. The one small act of switching hands will prove to be a general nuisance. (BTW- be sure to wear your least favorite watch when you try this!)

Second, both of these stories depended upon an expert: someone with an understanding of what was wrong, and who used their knowledge to fix the situation. I believe that by the time you get through reading this book you will know which little things are contributing to your pain, and with some thought you will know *decisively* what you need to do about it. (As a side benefit, many of the suggestions I wish to impart to you can improve your overall quality of life, regardless of whether or not you actually have any back issues.) I want you to be the expert. It's time for you to become the agent for your own wellness, and become your own guru.

With this in mind, it's time to leave your home, and venture out into the world.

The morning commute...

For a time, in an earlier part of my career, I had an hour-and-a-half commute each way to and from my office. My first job out of residency was in the middle of *Bumblesburg* (just East of *Nowhere*), and I had a drive consisting of about 45 minutes on the highway, followed by another 30-45 minutes (depending upon the weather) on narrow mountain roads. Pretty much every person I spoke to had the same question: *'Doesn't that destroy your back?'* Thankfully, no I didn't destroy my back- but it was largely because I anticipated the likelihood that this could be a problem, and was proactive in taking steps to make sure I eliminated as many of the anatomic bombs as

I could, and remained ok. With some forethought, even the longest drive can be a pain-free experience.

Many of us spend at least a part of our day in a car, and even with a short commute, you may be putting yourself at risk for problems. From a body mechanics standpoint, a car is one of the worst possible places. In a car, your lumbar spine remains in a flexed position, placing tension on exactly the portion of the vertebral disc most likely to herniate. If you are driving, your arms extend out in front of you, putting stress on your upper back and neck. To make matters worse, for the majority of your time in a car, you simply *don't move,* and, I always say: *if you rest, you rust.* Our bodies simply hate not moving. So many patients tell me that a ride in the car, long or short, leaves them feeling stiff and sore, and in some cases- utterly miserable. It's not because car manufacturers aren't trying --today's cars are so much better for your back than they were even ten or fifteen years ago-- but given the ergonomic problems inherent to driving, there's only so much they can do. Even the most expensive luxury cars still lack in this department. Despite the manufacturer's best efforts, there is no real way to make a car truly back-friendly. However, a little effort on your part can dramatically improve your odds of arriving at your destination unscathed.

Here are some simple suggestions for pain-free motoring:

Adjust: Before you start on your journey, check your reach, both to the pedals and to the steering wheel. Adjust your seat so your arms don't extend straight out, and yet don't bend too sharply at the elbows. Your legs should extend out in front of you so that your knees don't fall outwards (This puts strain on your hips which over time will cause your hip flexor muscles to become tight and alter your body mechanics, both while you are still seated, and more so once you get out of your car). If you are purchasing a new car (or a new used car) try to find one that has both an adjustable seat *and* steering wheel. This will provide you with the most opportunity to adjust for a good balance for driving comfort. Experiment with different positions to find the best possible location.

Check your view: Adjust your mirrors. Back in driver's ed. you learned how to do this before you begin your trip for clear views of the road, but if you are like most people, you're probably doing it wrong. Adjust rear and side view mirrors such that your neck is in a comfortable, neutral position while driving; you shouldn't have to change the position of your head when switching from the rear-view to the side-view mirror. This is not to say that you want to be immobile while driving, but rather that you not be uncomfortably extending your neck in one direction or another to see what's going on.

Move: When you are stopped at a light for a few moments, turn your head in opposite directions as far as you are comfortable. Do this several times to help prevent stiffness. Periodically, take your hands off the wheel. (Again, only while stopped!!! I can hear it now- *"But your honor, Dr. Kirschner told me to."*), and extend your hands straight out in front of you towards the windshield. Stretch out your shoulders and upper back. Put your hands on the top of your head and extend your elbows backwards to help mobilize your upper back. By mobilizing the segments of your spine and preventing stiffness from setting in, these few simple range-of-motion exercises can make a huge difference in how you feel once you arrive at your destination.

Breathe: At lights, take a moment for 2-3 deep

cleansing breaths to mobilize your spine, and get good aeration of your lungs. Oxygen is *always* a good thing.

Support: If your car has inadequate support (like most), roll up a small towel or t-shirt to use as a lumbar support. Place it in the small of your back to help maintain a normal lumbar curve. Whatever you use as a support should not press your low back outward, but rather fill in the space in the small of your back to keep the lumbar curvature from flattening out when seated.

Hydrate: Stay hydrated: Water keeps your tissues lubricated. This tip is particularly useful for long car trips as continual hydration will of course have the added benefit of forcing you to periodically get out of the car so you can...

Stretch! : During longer drives, get out of the car and stretch every hour or so. Sure, you're in a rush to get where you are going -- but what's the point of traveling if you're going to arrive in pain? Wally World will still be there, even if you get there ten or fifteen minutes later- unless of course the park is closed so they can clean and renovate America's favorite family fun park. Uh huh! (My references become more obscure as this book continues. Good grief, I miss John Candy.)

These tips should help you to arrive pain-free.

The power of breathing...

Twice already, I have recommended breathing exercises as part of your routine, so this is probably a good time to share some thoughts on the importance of quality breathing. You've breathed your whole life- but how many times have you given any thought to precisely *how* you breathe?

Individuals in pain will often exchange their regular smooth breathing patterns for jagged, short, shallow breaths, which can leave them feeling even more uncomfortable. I cannot overstate the benefits of good breathing patterns towards your general state of wellness. Nearly as useful as quality sleep, deep cleansing breaths do several important things:

Oxygenate: Deep breaths more efficiently deliver needed oxygen to your tissues.

Mobilize: Like any other muscles in your body, the intercostal muscles- the narrow muscles in between your ribs- can become tight when they are underutilized; deep breaths are equivalent to a range of motion exercise for these key muscles. Deep inhalation will move ribs, thoracic and lumbar vertebrae, loosening up structures and encouraging normal thoracic function.

Heal: Deep inspiration stimulates a portion of the lymphatic system known as the thoracic duct, helping to move cellular waste products and other toxins out of your body. Cleansing breaths can make you feel healthier, and in theory, help you to heal more quickly. I recommend doing several sessions of deep breaths throughout the day.

While you may think you've gotten a pretty good handle on breathing, here is a simple approach to taking deep cleansing breaths:

-Stand with your legs a little wider than shoulder width apart (while you can do them seated if need be, being seated will restrict the full movement of your diaphragm making the exercise somewhat less effective). Take a slow deep breath through your nose, filling your lungs as much as you can. When you think they are full- try to take in just a little more and hold it for five to seven seconds.

-Slowly exhale your breath through pursed lips until you feel there is nothing left.

-When it feels like there's no air left, puff the last little bit of breath out through your lips, and then repeat the whole process 3-4 times in a row, several times a day.

Taking time out of your day for some breathing exercises is definitively amongst the most important suggestions I will share with you, so take it seriously- you will be surprised at the difference this makes.

One of the reasons I thought this would be a great time to discuss breathing is because one of my favourite times to do deep breathing exercises is when I have first arrived at my office, before I begin my work for the day. The breathing exercises help me to feel energized, better able to cope with any of the stress I know will be headed my way, and get me ready to begin my work day.

Time for work...

I understand that not everyone works in an office, but the tips I am about to give you apply to your home office or the place you have your computer set up as well, so there is probably some place in your life where these suggestions apply.

I do workplace assessments all the time, and I am always amazed at how poorly some people set up their desks. Even things that should be obvious seem to be overlooked- it sometimes feels as though these workspaces are *designed* to cause back problems. For me, the fun thing about doing this type of assessment is the extent to which people are blown away at how much better they can feel at work by engaging in a few, simple changes. The best part is that it makes me look really smart to boot!

It is easy to spend lots of time sitting at a desk, browsing the internet, or even paying the bills, without paying attention to how the layout of this space could be affecting you. Here are some basic guidelines for setting up your workspace:

Computer monitor: Make sure your computer monitor is as close to eye level as possible, and that it is in front of you- not off to the side. When your neck is flexed, extended, or rotated left or right for prolonged periods, the muscles you use to hold the position get fatigued and can become stiff or sore. A neutral position will help to prevent this problem. You don't necessarily need to spend a ton of money on a monitor stand or new workstation furniture. You can prop your monitor up on old phone books, or any other stable surface- keeping your neck in a safer position, and with the monitor at a distance (not too close, not to far away) that will not force you to strain your eyes.

Keyboard: Keep your keyboard and mouse on the desk directly in front of the monitor and at a level that allows you to keep your forearm and wrist in a neutral position. Your wrist and forearm should rest parallel to the desktop, and your elbows should be in a relaxed position, not spread far from your body or uncomfortably close together. In this case, a non-neutral position places strain on your arms and shoulders, which will affect your upper back.

Desk chair: Get a desk chair with adequate lumbar support (again, a tightly rolled up t-shirt or small towel placed behind the small of your back will work in a pinch). Make certain that the seat is long enough from front to back that it supports your thighs- but not so long that you cannot comfortably rest your feet on the floor. Supporting your thighs will take strain off of your hips by disengaging the muscles that stabilize them.

-Adjust the height of your seat so your upper thighs are parallel to the floor with your toes lightly on the ground- you don't want your legs hanging off the edge of the chair, nor do you want your knees bent up towards your chest. Here, a neutral position will keep your hip abductor and adductor muscles from becoming fatigued. If your chair has armrests, make sure that they can fit underneath your desktop, otherwise they will keep your chair too far from your workspace, and force you to lean forward while you work.

Desk items: Keep the items you use the most in close proximity so you can avoid having to reach all over the place to get to them. This leaves my desk looking pretty cluttered, but at least my back feels great.

Hydrate!: As with any activity, remember to hydrate. Getting absorbed in their work can cause some people to overlook the need for water. Tanking up will again provide the added benefit of forcing you to...

Move: Get up every half hour or so. If you don't wear a watch, keep a clock nearby to remind you- or better yet, there are a whole bunch of downloadable freeware programs for your computer that will allow you to set an interval alarm. Remember, in a seated position your back is in flexion -- the position, which puts your low back most at risk. Periodically, you've got to get out of your chair and reach for the sky with a brief stretch- extending your back, and keeping things moving.

CRITICAL: And lastly but perhaps most importantly,

obtain a headset for your telephone. This is a serious pet peeve of mine. Having your phone wedged in between your ear and your shoulder is just asking for neck problems. If you hold your phone this way, it will make you hurt- maybe not today, maybe not tomorrow, but it will eventually catch up with you and cause you pain. Decent headsets can be had at your local electronics store for under ten bucks, so honestly there is really no excuse. I've seen even cheaper ones as low as $2.99 at my local convenience store.

Once again, since this is a place you are likely to spend a good deal of your time, you must give it the attention it deserves. A well-sorted workspace will provide many rewards, and further diminish the risk of contributing to your back issues.

Small things revisited...

Remember earlier when I said that *anything* and *everything* was a potential cause of your back pain? Here's another example of a surprising, apparently unrelated small thing having a profound effect on back pain:

I was evaluating a new patient who had developed back and neck pain over the previous several months. She had no injury or trauma that could account for her discomfort. We reviewed her x-rays, and they looked pretty normal for someone her age. She related that the pain only occurred when she was sitting at her computer. Immediately, we began to discuss any and all of the issues associated with her workspace. She adjusted the height of her monitor, even got a new (seriously expensive) desk chair with good support, and in spite of all of these efforts, she still had pain while working. I was able to correct the dysfunction in her spine with osteopathic treatment and she always left my office pain free. Still, in just a matter of days, she would call to set up another appointment. Frustrated, I finally set up a time to visit her office (this is not my standard method of doing things, but this case was driving me crazy- I thought I had left no stone unturned, and yet I still had no clear cause for her pain.) I got there and began to look at things first hand. As I looked around, everything was in order- she had done a great job of setting up an efficient and safe workspace, but was still hurting despite all of our efforts. Things became clear when I asked her to sit down and work. What I observed was that she had her head leaned in over her keyboard to better see her computer monitor- she couldn't focus on the screen if her head was more than a foot or so away from the screen.

"Susan, when did your pain actually start?"

"I would say, about four months ago." she replied.

"And when did you get those glasses?"

"Five months ago."

It turns out that Susan had recently had an eye exam and, for the first time in years she had had a significant change in her eyeglass prescription. While her ophthalmologist had gotten the prescription correct, her optician had not. It was close, but deviated enough that in order to compensate, Susan had to significantly alter her posture just to see the screen. To most observers, this change might have seemed subtle or even un-noticeable, but hey, I was running out of directions to take this. After observing her straining to see her monitor, I instructed her to return to her optician. It turned out that simply correcting her prescription solved her problem, and her back pain was gone. Really gone. Oh, and as an added bonus- she could see too!

Now, I have to say that in nearly two decades of thinking about these issues and treating literally thousands of patients, a bad eyeglass prescription had never been the cause of back pain before or since Susan's difficult experience (although I do see eyeglasses causing headaches quite frequently.) What this cautionary tale illustrates, once again, is that even the smallest, seemingly unrelated factor can cause back pain. In retrospect, her experience wasn't *all* bad, or at least it ended well; her back pain is gone, she can see, and her desk is finally set up correctly.

But I don't work at a desk...

I started this work section with desk ergonomics because even those who don't work from a desk likely have a desk space at home from where they manage their home-paying bills, scheduling things, even just to browse the Internet. So I felt the tips applied to most of you. But what if, like me, you don't do most of your work from a desk? What if you use your body for your living? I spend most of my day on my feet, leaning over patients, moving people's body parts all over the place (People don't realize how physical my work is until they get on my table. Often times, both my patients and I have worked up a pretty good sweat by the time I've completed their treatment.)

If your work is physical- and it doesn't matter if you are a physician, an assembly line worker, a landscaper, *whatever-* you have some unique considerations when trying to adjust for a back-friendly approach to work.

Everyone's work situation is unique. There's no real way within the scope of this book for me to get into all of the varied ergonomic conditions that exist in all of the different workplaces out there. But no matter what your unique circumstances are, there are some suggestions that are universal.

Prepare for your work.

Earlier, I told you that I begin my workday with a few deep cleansing breaths to help get my head clear and oxygen flowing out into my body. Take a few additional moments to loosen up; stiff joints and tight muscles can compromise your body mechanics and set you up for injury. This situation can be worsened if you had a long commute to work and didn't take steps to keep yourself out of trouble, as outlined in the section on commuting. A good, general-purpose, pre-work stretch routine looks a little like this:

1) Take three slow deep breaths. As you inhale with your third, raise your hands over your head reaching as far up as you can towards the ceiling. This will help open up the shoulder girdle, and mobilize your rib cage. Hold this for 5-10 seconds.

2) As you exhale this breath, lower your outstretched arms out in front of you, spreading your fingers apart, and rounding your shoulders towards your outstretched arms. This will help to loosen up the upper thoracic spine. Hold this position for 5-10 seconds.

3) Allow your arms to drop to your sides and slowly rotate your head in each direction, holding it for a few seconds at the end of each rotation. As you repeat this rotation, try to add a few extra degrees at the end of your range each time. This frees up the movement of your neck. Do three repetitions per side.

4) Cross your arms in front of you, and with your feet slightly wider than shoulder width apart, slowly rotate your upper body to the both sides to the end-range-of-motion- again adding a couple of extra degrees of rotation with each repetition. This stretch helps mobilize the lower thoracic and upper lumbar spine, and elongates some of the rotator muscles as well. Do three repetitions per side.

5) Place the palms of your hands on the front of your thighs, and slowly slide your hands down your thighs as far as you can comfortably go. When you get to the end

range, hold it for 5-10 seconds, then slowly come back up to a neutral, standing position. Do not bounce! This helps mobilize the lower lumbar spine, and elongates the three larger muscles running up each side of your spine. It will also help loosen the hamstrings. Do three repetitions per side.

6) Move your hands to the sides of your thighs, and slide your right hand down your right thigh, going down as far as you comfortably can, holding it for 5-10 seconds, then change sides. This stretch will help lengthen the paraspinal muscles, as well as mobilize the lumbar & thoracic spinal segments and rib cage. Do three repetitions per side.

7) Using a wall or table/desktop as support, slowly raise your body onto your tiptoes. Hold this position for a few seconds. This mobilizes the joints in your feet and ankles,

and gently stretches the gastrocnemius muscles of your calves. Do three repetitions.

8) Extend one leg straight behind you, placing both of your hands on your bent knee in front of you. Slowly press backwards into your back heel. As you hold this stretch, gently rotate your upper body in the direction *opposite* the extended leg (i.e.- If your left leg is extended behind you, rotate your upper torso to the right). Hold this position for approximately 10 seconds. This stretch simultaneously further elongates the calf muscles, and the iliopsoas muscle (tightness in the iliopsoas is a common cause of low back discomfort.) Do 2 repetitions per side.

9) Close with three more deep cleansing breaths.

This whole preventive routine should take you less than five minutes, and can help keep you pain-free throughout the day. Again, please keep in mind that this should be considered a general-purpose stretch. You may find that additional and replacement stretches could more appropriately prepare you for your kind of work. The take-home message is that preparation is the most effective measure of prevention- so take the time to stretch.

The coffee break walk...

I sometimes find that I may have a cancellation, or a patient no-show, or some other part of my day where I'm not working for a few moments. For you, it could be lunchtime or during a coffee break. I look to these times of my day as an opportunity to get out and move for a while. Whenever I have those moments, I put on a pair of headphones and take a walk around the block, giving me a chance to stretch out my legs and clear my head. Be sure to add a few breaths at the beginning of your walk, in order to get the most of this mini-workout. This can be useful whether you have five minutes, or a whole lunch hour (of course, don't skip lunch.) This simple activity can transform your day by mobilizing your whole body, and keeping you from getting stiff. As an added bonus you'll also burn a few calories!

Managing YOU...

You've already heard me allude to the psychological component of pain, and for many reasons, this can be the most difficult part of the trapezoid to address. If you've been suffering with back or neck pain, you already know that it affects everything you do. In fact, it may have already begun to take its toll on others around you-particularly family members or coworkers. When pain goes on for a while, it can cause problems emotionally as well as physically. When it goes on longer than that, the challenge is to prevent pain from becoming part of your identity- part of who you are- where it can then go on to reap even more significant and hard-to-correct problems.

In my practice, I explain to patients the distinction between a *person who is sick* and a *sick person*. This sounds like a subtle difference, but it really isn't.

Imagine two people with the same low back pain: The person who is sick wakes up in the morning and says *'It is sure going to be tough to do the things I need to do because I don't feel well.'* Conversely, the sick person says *'I won't be able to do the things I need to do because I don't feel well.'* Now I know everybody has a different pain tolerance- but this goes beyond the notion of tolerance- this difference gets at the very heart of *who you are.*

How do you avoid the trap of becoming a sick person? How does one manage a semblance of optimism when dealing with ongoing pain? One of the most effective suggestions I have found is this: *You need to take time for yourself.*

This may sound self-evident, but in today's busy world, with long work hours, family obligations, and an ever-expanding list of responsibilities, it can be very easy to forget to take care of yourself and give yourself the time you need. I divide this time into three distinct parts (which allows me to once again have a *triad*! Woo hoo!!!)

The *You* Management Triad

Rest

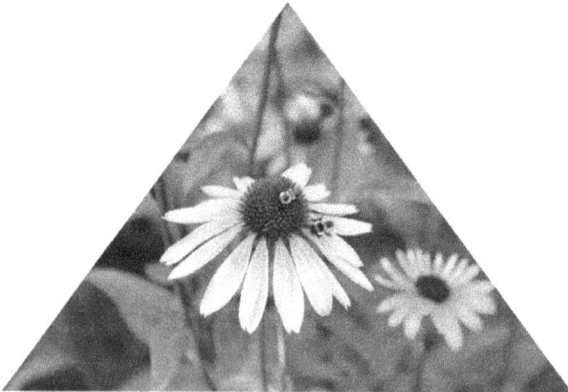

Recreation   Reflection

Rest: We've already discussed the importance of sleep. Without quality rest, nothing else you do is going to help much to reduce your pain- hence its position at the top of the triad. GET SLEEP! GET SLEEP! GET SLEEP! There's just no way to overstate the importance of this. Furthermore, when it is sensible to do so, give yourself some protected pockets of 'down time' throughout your day. Physical and emotional fatigue will only exacerbate your problems. Chill!

Recreation: How do you relax and have fun? Some people give up on their hobbies or retreat from their social lives when confronted with back pain- which is a really bad idea. These activities keep you from focusing on your pain, and continue to help restore normalcy to a life which may otherwise feel compromised by the ever-present specter of pain. Additionally, this can be the area where your loved ones begin to suffer because of *you* and your condition as they start to lose out on experiences and activities they would previously have shared with you. In many relationships, this leaves partners feeling like that's a situation they didn't sign up for. Consider the activities you do for recreation. Are there things you've given up since you began to experience pain? Are there things you could potentially be doing that would not exacerbate your discomfort? When you have identified these activities, slowly reintroduce some of them into your life. It may take some time for your body to become re-acclimated to the more physical activities you've given up, so don't become frustrated if you find yourself sore at first- this is normal and will be a part of the healing process. For peace of mind, you can consult your physician if you are concerned these activities might potentially cause you further injury. If you have been previously doing these activities with a loved one, be sure to invite them to share in your recovery and join you. This can help you to heal both your pain and your relationship!

Reflection: First off- this is *not* your time to reflect on just how awful you feel. No. This is your quiet time of the day- a time to consider all of the things in your life that are going *well*, and to feel gratitude for all of them. This is also a time to focus on those times throughout your life when perhaps your pain is not as bad as other times. When I consider time for reflection, I often think back to something my wife (a natural childbirth instructor, who God bless her, gave birth to both of our children without any pain medications), said to me one time when she saw me suffering with a particularly large kidney stone- a condition known for its horrible pain. I had been in terrible pain continuously for about 3 days, in a burgeoning state of panic due to my inability to function at even a rudimentary level, when she calmly said to me 'There are times in your life you will feel pain, and most of the other times when you don't. This is temporary, and will get better. Try to mentally latch onto the times you are feeling good."

What insightful advice! Whenever we are in pain, we tend to focus on the discomfort, and how bad we feel right now. In truth, it is much more useful to latch onto the times you feel good (or latch on to the notion of an outcome, as when dealing with the pain of childbirth.) When in your day do you feel good? Is there any part of the day when you at least feel a little *better?* When was the last time you felt *great?*

If you need proof that your psychology directly affects your physiology, try this simple exercise. Close your eyes for a few moments, and focus on one of these examples (if *none* of these examples applies to you then (a) you are very lucky and (b) you're going to have to focus on something else- try to think of something that's equally terrible!):

-Breaking up with a boyfriend/girlfriend when you were in high school.

-A terrible fight you had with a parent or spouse.

-Getting fired from a job.

-Try this one: how about the last time you missed something special you wanted to do because of your back pain?

As you focus on these experiences, really try to relive them in your mind. Mentally go back to where you were emotionally when these things actually occurred. Heck, you probably replayed them a thousand times already right after they actually occurred- trying to formulate how you would have handled things differently. As you focus on these experiences, you may notice your body tensing up, your breaths becoming more shallow, and perhaps even any pain you may be experiencing at that moment getting worse. Now I have no intention of keeping you in this bad place for long. Let's take you away from these bad feelings and bring you to a place where you felt better. Try to refocus on one of these examples:

-Your first kiss.

-Graduation.

-Your wedding day.

-Winning 'The Big Game.' **

-Focusing on all of the things you look forward to being able to do once you are out of pain.

** In years of doing this exercise with patients, both in my practice, and in live seminars, I've never encountered anyone who actually won 'the Big Game.' I know you're out there somewhere- shoot me an email and share your experience with me.

As you focus on these more positive examples- again, really aiming to re-live them in your mind, you may notice a profound sense of relaxation washing over your body. The tension in your shoulders will begin to diminish, your breaths may slow down and become deeper, and your pain may start to improve. Aim for this state during your periods of reflection; it is a necessary component of the pain-free lifestyle.

Focusing on the pain can keep you trapped in the mindset of feeling bad. Thinking about the times in your life when you felt good, or even anticipating the future when you might be feeling better, can be one of the most powerful tools for reducing and ultimately recovering from pain.

As you deal with pain, take time in your day to reflect upon the times when you feel good. When are the times of your day or week when you don't feel quite as bad?

Perhaps they are during time spent with a loved one, or listening to music- it really doesn't matter what- these are the times you should focus on. Visualize yourself feeling great, and look forward to that time when you will feel better than you do now. It may be hard when in the throes of serious discomfort, but with concentration and focus, these periods of meditation will help you to feel less pain in the now, and to ultimately recover faster. You probably have already noticed how much your mood affects your pain- this is a tool you can use to help guide a useful change in your mood and your physiology.

No matter how busy your life is, it is absolutely imperative that you set aside time for yourself to attend to all three aspects of the triad *every single day for the rest of your life* It doesn't necessarily need to be a long period of time to be effective either. A few minutes can be all that's needed to do the trick (By the way- this is also a great time to do some of the breathing exercises we discussed before.) You can feel free to fold some of the recreation and reflection time into each other- particularly if you use some form of exercise as recreation. I find that one of the best opportunities I have to clear my head is when I am out on the trails on my mountain bike. What are yours?

At first, some people feel selfish designating this special time for themselves during the course of a hectic day, particularly if they are an individual imbued with the responsibility of caring for others. Let me reassure you *that this is an instance where you are allowed to be selfish.* Got that? From this modest fit of selfishness, you will feel better, and ultimately do a better job caring for everyone else. Defend this time of your day as vigorously as you would defend your sleep- it's that important.

What's cooking?: *Creating your back-friendly kitchen.*

We were having dinner with our friends, Sandra and Dave. I watched as our hosts ran back and forth in their kitchen preparing our meal. I marveled at all of the anatomic bombs I noticed throughout the kitchen while the two of them cooked. I hesitated to broach the topic, as they had just spent an inordinate amount of cash renovating their kitchen. Absolutely beautiful, the space was an ergonomic and anatomic disaster area! After dinner, Donna and I helped to clear the table, and as Dave stood behind the sink taking our dishes, I noticed him rubbing his own back, and trying to nonchalantly do some little sidebending stretches. I saw this as my entree to the discussion about the problems I saw lurking in their kitchen.

"How's your back, Dave?"

"Its a little sore, but I'll be ok." he replied.

"Does that happen to you a lot when you cook?"

"Only when we make a big meal."

"I was kind of noticing some things about the setup of your kitchen as you were cooking, and I really think there are a few things you could move around which could really help you and Sandy to have a better time while cooking- particularly with your back."

Dave looked at me incredulously, tilting his head to the side a little, and paused.

"You know, Sandra and I spent a lot of time designing this kitchen, and making sure the layout made sense. We worked with a great designer who helped us work the whole thing through. I doubt you could really do much to improve it- you're a doctor not an interior designer," he tersely noted.

At this point Sandra chimed in "*I sometimes get a sore back when I'm cooking- do you honestly think you can change things without having to tear down the whole thing and start from scratch?"*

We cracked open a bottle of wine, and set about addressing some of my concerns, moved a bunch of things around, and came up with a short list of items they needed to purchase. The entire time, Dave seemed seriously annoyed with the whole process- after all, he had hired *Pierre- The Kitchen Expert* to set up his kitchen- what could I possibly have to contribute? When we finished, I said to Dave, "*Look, do these things for a few weeks, and see if they make a difference. If they don't, fine, I'm wrong- I'll cook you dinner, and serve an amazing bottle of Port. But if in the end they help you'll be thanking me- and I'm gonna put your story in my next book- and you'll be buying the Port."*

I didn't hear from Dave or Sandy for several weeks after I had called them the following day to thank them for the lovely dinner. Perhaps I really had offended them? One afternoon, Donna called me to tell me that we had been invited to dinner at their home the following Friday. Well, we were enthusiastically greeted when we arrived.

"Andy, I'm a schmuck" Dave exclaimed while handing me a glass of Vintage Port (my friends all know how much I love good Port- and now so do you. After your back pain goes away, you'll know what to send me! I prefer 77's and 85's) *"You were right. I was wrong. As much as I liked my kitchen after the renovations, now I love it."*

My work there was done. Reputation maintained. Honor restored. **IN YOUR FACE PIERRE!!**

So, how can your kitchen cause you back problems? Well, if you think about it, your kitchen is not all that different from a factory assembly line, and like any workplace, you can set yourself up for injury through poor ergonomics and repetitive stress. Also, like any workplace, some thoughtful attention to the layout and workflow can help reduce the risk. Consider these suggestions:

Arrange your kitchen work areas by activity.

Place your cutting and chopping items near the area you would likely place your cutting board to chop vegetables, cleaning items near the sink, pots and pans close to the stove, etc. This will keep you from running back and forth unnecessarily, and decrease your amount of repetitive stress.

Put pots and pans on an overhead rack.

Get a hanging pot rack, and install it near your stove, not

so high up that you need to reach uncomfortably to get them. Keeping your pots and pans, particularly those that weigh the most, in a low cabinet, puts your back at risk every time you bend deeply to reach for them. In our kitchen, we placed a rigidly mounted shelf over our stove to hold our cast iron cookery. If you have an infrequently used back burner on your stove, you can nest a couple of the larger pots there. Hang the pot lids on the wall directly over the stove.

Get a barstool with wheels to sit on for longer tasks. If you've just served a large dinner, standing in front of the sink for an hour cleaning dishes will do your back no favors, as the muscles of the lumbar spine are likely already fatigued. The same thing also applies if you need to spend a long time chopping or cutting items. An adjustable-height rolling bench will provide you the same benefit when performing lower-

down tasks such as oven cleaning. I prefer stools with backs- you then have the option of adding some lumbar support.

If you are using a dishwasher, put the silverware basket in the sink and load and unload utensils all at once to minimize repetitive movement. To reach, turn, and put items away into the drawer -- over and over -- is exactly the same as the repetitive movements ergonomic experts have worked so hard to eliminate in factories and manufacturing facilities. Also, use a pull-out organizer for your silverware drawer so you can place the basket from the dishwasher and the organizer for your drawer next to each other, and reduce your twisting and bending even more.

Keep some simple kitchen cleaning items on the counter next to your sink- perhaps some smaller containers with smaller amounts of cleaners and soap that are easier to handle than the large economy bottles. This way you won't constantly reach underneath and into the cabinet to get to frequently used items.

Place the heavier items in your refrigerator on higher shelves when possible, to reduce the amount of stressful bending you'll have to do. Some refrigerators do not have high shelves that can easily support heavier items, such as a turkey- so do the best you can, parting things out into smaller, more manageable containers. Gallons of milk should either be kept high, or partially emptied into a smaller serving container. For the lower shelves, try to group similar items into easily pulled organizing baskets (cheeses in one, condiments in one, etc.) This will make retrieving all of these items easier on your back.

Plan your kitchen activities ahead of time. If you will be preparing a large meal, or one with multiple ingredients, requiring many utensils- take them out ahead of time and organize your workspace accordingly, perhaps thinking about your upcoming meal preparation as a timeline- laying out what you need in order across the countertop.

Now here's the expensive one; get a stress mat for each of your work areas.

Many on-line retailers sell these shock absorbing mats, that help absorb some of the stress and impact from standing in one spot, protect your feet, and ultimately help protect your back. My home has a small kitchen, so one four by six foot mat pretty much does the job- but I've been in kitchens where several mats were needed- one in front of the sink, one for the stove, one for the prep area. Wherever you spend time on your feet in the kitchen, that's where you need them.

Food always tastes better when you are not in pain. Now get yourself back into the kitchen, and *start cooking!*

Clean up time...

I just gave you a few simple suggestions for straightening out your kitchen, but one of the most back stressing activities for many people is housecleaning. Even a small apartment can represent a veritable minefield of anatomic bombs just waiting to ruin your day.

As with any routine task, there are a few things you can do to help get things straight, and keep you out of pain. Try some of these tips to help keep your house clean, and your back pain-free:

Prepare your mind and body for the task. As with any other physical activity, preparing your body can prevent injury. Take a moment to gently stretch out, and as you do so, think about your tasks ahead, and consider the order in which you will proceed in an effort to decrease the amount of stress to which you will be subjecting your body. And, as always, hydrate before, during, and after.

Divide and conquer. You may have gotten into the habit of assigning a single day for your housecleaning tasks. A better suggestion is to divide up your home into more manageable sections, and do a little each day to prevent yourself from 'overdoing it' on any given day.

Organize. Some people keep a bucket of cleaning supplies, and mops and brooms in a closet somewhere in their home, and pull them out and drag them all over the house when going from room to room. A better suggestion, particularly in homes with more than one floor, is to get a small basket or bucket, and keep a small annex of cleaning supplies for each region of the house- along with a broom or mop on each floor. If you are really committed to this, you could even purchase a smaller, lighter vacuum cleaner for each floor rather than the industrial strength one you may be using for the whole house (This is one area where manufacturers have really stepped up their game. There are quality lightweight vacuums available at almost any price point.)

Declutter on the fly. Entropy is real! It is remarkable how quickly messes will accumulate- particularly if you live with kids. Try to get into the habit (and *gently* encourage those you live with as well) of picking things up, and putting them away as you finish with them. We all have the *intention* of doing this, but in practice, most people don't. This tip has a twofold benefit: First, you will be dividing up a task, which could rapidly become overwhelming. Second, you will decrease the likelihood of tripping over something and sustaining a fall that would only make your back problems worse.

Clean up your cleanup. Some will argue that this is not specifically a back-pain-related tip, but in my experience it is. Many household cleaners contain caustic chemicals, which are irritating to the skin and breathing passages. The less exposed to these harsh chemicals you find yourself, the better off you will be. Try to find safer organic alternatives to cleaning products when possible (You won't believe how clean simple white vinegar can make things!) Additionally, clean your cleaning stuff- all of your tools can get dusty and covered with residue, which can further contribute to your feeling lousy. Put on an inexpensive dust mask, and clean it all off.

Time with the kids...

Pretty much everyone who carries kids frequently, be it parents, grandparents, aunts, uncles- whoever- has dealt with some discomfort as a result. In my own experience as a parent, the more tired and wiped out I was from the activities of my day, the more likely it was that my kids wanted or needed to be picked up. In my practice, the folks most likely to have back problems as a result of carrying kids are almost always the parents of newborns- particularly parents with a *first child* (I will get to why that makes a difference in just a moment). Think about it based upon what you already know from reading this book: new parents have poor sleep and greatly increased levels of stress. They are performing activities they are not conditioned to do, including activities involving repetitive movements. Add to this the fact that they are schlepping around a whole lot of heavy stuff: The baby, diaper bag, changing mat, toys, car seat, brain-enhancing DVDs, nursing pillow, soothing baby sounds portable radio, bouncy seat, change of clothes, and all of the other (often unnecessary) paraphernalia associated with having a new baby- all of which weigh about six hundred pounds. Being a new parent is essentially the trifecta of back pain.

The reason I say that back issues are more common with new parents of a first child is that parents of a second child have typically gotten smart- and they leave a lot of this unnecessary crap at home! Interestingly, postpartum women are at greater risk than many, largely because of the physiology of pregnancy: women typically gain weight during their pregnancy at a higher rate than at any other time in their lives, the majority of which placed at exactly the location where it could do the most damage to the lumbar spine. Combine this with the fact that pregnant women produce a hormone known as *relaxin* (not *relaxin'*), which helps to loosen up the ligaments and connective tissue through the pelvis- opening the birth canal, making it easier for a baby to pass through. Unfortunately, relaxin is indiscriminate- it doesn't just loosen up the ligaments around the pelvis- it loosens up *everything-* potentially destabilizing the whole musculoskeletal system. This combination of factors is why such a disproportionate number of pregnant women develop back pain. In spite of this 'perfect storm' setup, back pain does not need to be an inevitability, either for pregnant women *or* for new parents.

Tips for pregnant women:

As always, defend your sleep. We've already covered this, but it bears repetition. In addition to the weight gain and hormonal changes, a pregnant woman's body is very metabolically active- quality sleep is essential to allow her body to recharge and recover.

Sleep in the correct position. Pregnant women are often asked not to sleep on their backs, but rather to sleep on their left side. When on your side, extend the top leg forward, stabilizing your body, and taking some pressure off of your lumbar spine. In the Osteopathic world, this is known as the *Modified Simms Position,* and is often used as a pre-treatment position prior to having spinal adjustments performed. You can enhance the stability of this position by placing a small pillow between your knees. This will help prevent you from rolling forward while you sleep, and help to keep your hips in a neutral position. Many pregnant women enjoy snoozing with a body pillow, which supports their bellies as well.

Do some gentle stretching. While relaxin helps to loosen connective tissue, this is often countered by tightening up of the muscles of the low back, hips and pelvis. Take some time, several times a day, to stretch out these fatigued muscles. Even better, try some prenatal yoga to help keep things moving the way they are supposed to.

Tips for New parents:

Lose the baby bucket. The convertible baby car seats that also serve as a baby carrier *look* like they're a great convenience, but in truth, they are an anatomic bomb of the first order. They weigh a lot, and in spite of how designers try to make the handles more ergonomic- they are all well and truly awful. Baby buckets place the bulk of the baby's weight off of the parents' center of gravity, forcing them to lean to one side or the other.

If for some peculiar reason you feel you *need* to carry one of these ergonomic time bombs, be sure to switch sides and take breaks often. That's pretty much all that can be done here. In my opinion, a better option would be to leave the baby carrier in the car, where it likely excels as a car seat and then...

Try a baby sling or close-body baby carrier. Baby slings have several advantages over the baby bucket. They weigh pretty much nothing. They keep your baby's weight close to your center of gravity. Slings bring your baby closer to your eye level, giving you a better view of them, and giving them better opportunity to interact with you and be stimulated by the world at large. They are a huge convenience for nursing mothers, offering a supportive platform (and a simple way to preserve modesty if you feel like you need to!) They are easy to wash when your baby pukes on it (or worse!- and believe me- this will happen to your sling and your car seat- but it's a lot harder to throw your car seat in the washing machine!) There are just so many reasons why this is a better option. It may take a week or so for most

parents to get used to using them, but they can make a world of difference.

Sit down. Rather than constantly carrying your child- for example while bouncing them to pacify them or help them fall asleep- get a good supportive chair to place near the place they sleep, and keep them on your lap. You can bounce them just as effectively on your knee.

Pare down. Remember that comprehensive list of baby-related crap I gave you at the beginning of the section? You pretty much don't need most of the items on that list. By the time my older daughter was about 3 months old, we managed to be able to leave the house with her in the baby sling, a couple of extra diapers and wipes tucked away in the bottom of the sling, and maybe a toy or two in the free hand. The flattened sling makes a great changing pad and works fine as a little place to rest when you have a chance to put your sleeping baby down. You will feel so much better, lighter, and more efficient leaving all the other stuff at home.

Nurse! I'm not going to get into all of the biological reasons why nursing is advantageous for your baby- just those that specifically pertain to your back pain. Nursing allows you to leave an entire additional set of items home, so you don't have to carry them. More importantly, nursing sends a chemical signal back to your body, telling it that your pregnancy has ended, causing a more rapid decline in the amount of relaxin being produced, thereby helping to re-stabilize the spine.

Some tips for pain-free nursing:

1) Nursing with your baby in a sling is easier on your back than trying to hold her in your arms.

2) Give your back a little rest- sit down to nurse.

3) Nursing pillows are great when you are at home, where you will likely be doing most of your nursing- but leave them home. It's just something else you have to carry around with you!

If you choose to bottle-feed your baby, try to switch the sides that you hold her for feedings from time to time.

Keeping your back safe from toddlers:

Toddlers bring an altogether different set of anatomic bombs. As much as parents seem to have back issues with newborn children, it is the grandparents who most often wind up in my office after chasing down toddlers. Even as kids grow and change over time, they still like to be picked up- sometimes for fun and sometimes to find comfort when they are upset. If you're like me, you can't say no- and in truth you wouldn't want to anyway. Some thoughts on wrangling toddlers, and remaining pain-free:

Get down! So much more can be accomplished with children when you are at eye level. Rather than picking up your child every time the need arises, try squatting down on your haunches, or better yet sit with them on your lap so you can speak with them face to face. This reduces the amount of time you will spend supporting their weight and in a bent / flexed position. Additionally, studies have shown that conferring with your kids at their eye level enhances their sense of wellbeing, which will ultimately make things a little easier for you.

Like it or not, you* will *pick them up. When you do, remember to use good lifting mechanics: bending at the knees and *not* with your back, carrying your child on your hip, and switching sides often. It is easy to forget to use correct lifting techniques, as you may have been accustomed to lifting wrong. A fun tip here is to ask your child of about 3 or older to remind you before you pick them up. Tell them it is an important job- they won't forget, believe me.

Control the mess. Having your children pick up after themselves from a young age is not just a good habit for them to develop, it will keep you from repetitively bending to pick things up, and decrease the likelihood that you will trip over a toy or other item which has been left out, fall, and leave yourself in even more discomfort.

Keeping your kids out of trouble...

A newer problem that I've been seeing of late, is something I thought *(Hoped!)* I would never see: *Kids with back pain.* Of all of the demographics out there, school age children really should be near the bottom of the pile in terms of likely-to-have-back-pain groups. Despite this, I am seeing it more and more, both in my practice, and in the medical literature. There are a several possible explanations for this:

Many kids are more sedentary than ever. Between school, and time spend on the internet/ in front of the TV/ playing video games, many kids are simply not as active as they need to be, which can lead to...

Obesity. The incidence of childhood obesity is on the rise, and this places strains on a child's back which just don't need to be there. On the other hand...

Many kids are totally overbooked, often with very physical activities. Multiple sports, clubs, and other after school activities can leave kids physically worn out, and with very little down time, contributing to the fact that...

Many kids are stressed out. School, after-school activities, sports, social activities, too much exposure to adult stresses and all of the other things kids have on their plates can leave kids feeling a lot of anxiety. Add to this the need to perform in school, and the competitive nature of it all makes kids feel stress. As I've said, stress in and of itself doesn't cause anything. It simply makes conditions you have *feel* worse.

It can be difficult enough to deal with back pain in adults, but it is just so hard to see young kids in pain. As parents, you can do a lot to prevent your children from hurting. Consider these suggestions:

Get them up and Get them out. Limit your child's screen time (TV, computer, tablet, or phone.) There is a certain amount of time needed for homework, and time with social media (But mom- ALL the kids are on Facebook!), but beyond that- get your kids up out of their seats and outside playing. As always, if you *rest* you *rust- and the only thing worse than a rusty parent, is a rusty kid!* Just as it does for you, prolonged sitting places your child's spine in a flexed position, placing stress on the paraspinal muscles and discs, putting them at risk for pain.

Empty the book bag. Earlier, I asked you to dump the contents of your purse or briefcase, and pare down the contents to just the things you actually need. Do the same for your kids. You wouldn't believe the things that you'll find going through your kid's book bags with them- lost clothing, missing homework assignments, uneaten lunches- all things that add up to your child schlepping around a lot more weight than they need to, fatiguing their muscles, and putting them at greater risk for injury.

Roll with it. No matter how much you clear out from their book bags, some kids are just burdened with too much weight from notebooks, textbooks, computers and other school necessities. If your child's school cannot provide an extra set of texts for your child to leave home (surprisingly many school districts _will_ make this accommodation) get your kids a rolling backpack so their spines do not need to support as much weight.

Now, if your kids are anything like mine, you'll be met with 'But I'll look like a dork!' Your obvious reply should be to counter with a question: Which looks dorkier? Using a rolling backpack, or walking around clutching your back, hunched over in the shape of a question mark? Regardless of whether this logic works for your child, you are the parent, and it's your responsibility to protect your kids from harm.

One of my favorite tips to give parents applies even more so as your kids grow. Kids get involved with any number of activities and sports (hopefully not *too* many simultaneously.) Tennis, soccer, gymnastics, mountain biking- there's just no end to the list of things your children may find interesting. As your child embarks upon these activities- try to involve yourself where and when it makes sense, participating in these activities. One of the nicer things that has happened in my family in the past several years was to discover that my daughter enjoys mountain biking- and now it's something we get to share with each other. This has been great for our relationship, gives us a chance to clear our heads together, and have some really great talks. Getting yourself out there to play a set of tennis, toss a frisbee or take a run every now and then- or whatever activities you share- will have the added benefit of getting *your* ass out the door and doing something beneficial for your body.

Hobbies...

Your interests and hobbies help your mental and social life. Recreation imbues our lives outside of work with meaning. My wife became an avid knitter after she finished her dissertation and needed to move away from the world of words for a while. While it's fed her soul, knitting became a strain on her eyes, neck and wrists. She now wears glasses for this close work, stretches out her neck every few rows and uses circular needles to reduce wrist fatigue. I urge you to assess your hobbies to see how you can address any lurking anatomic bombs. Here are a few suggestions for certain categories of hobbies:

Hobbies that require that we sit:

Handwork (knitting, crocheting, needlework), reading, model-building, puzzles, board games, tv-watching etc.

can strain eyes and necks. Be sure to look up and across the room or, better yet, out the window. This will take your neck out of a fixed position, and give your eyes the chance to adjust to different distances, or *focal lengths,* helping to relieve eyestrain. Take advantage of intermissions or the pause button on your DVD or DVR if you do these activities while watching television or movies. Get up every thirty to forty-five minutes to stretch out and give your back a break. Do neck rotations at regular intervals- every five rows, pages, during commercial breaks, etc.

Gardening: When the weather is right, I'm pretty much always out in my garden during my free time. There are few things more relaxing and rejuvenating than putting together the oasis in your backyard to help you escape the rigmarole of our hectic lives outside the home. Unfortunately, this calming activity can leave you stiff and sore if you don't take adequate steps to protect yourself. Try some of these tips for back-friendly gardening:

Mulching? Do small areas with a small pail or bag rather than hauling around a hundred pound bag and injuring yourself. For larger areas, a wheelbarrow is a must.

Don't be afraid to get a little dirty. Rather than bending over to pull weeks or plant flowers, find a spot and *sit down*. When you do need to bend, be sure to bend at the knees and *not* your back.

Plan your tasks ahead of time. Have all of your necessary items nearby, which will reduce the need to get up and down repeatedly. I keep my small gardening tools in a lightweight plastic bin with a handle, making it easier to move from one work area to the next.

When you purchase new garden tools, try to stick with tools with long handles, decreasing your need to bend and constantly get up and down.

Give yourself periodic breaks. It's easy to get involved in one task or another and lose track of time. Step back periodically and enjoy your progress, giving your body a chance to rest.

Lastly- as always - **_HYDRATE!_** Even a little dehydration can set you up for injury, or make any back pain you have even worse. Also, while this doesn't specifically pertain to back pain- always remember to use sunscreen and wear a broad-brimmed hat to protect yourself from harmful sun exposure.

These tips should help you to spend time enjoying your garden without pain!

Weekend warriors: As a general rule, be sure to use the correct, well maintained equipment for whatever sport you do. I can't tell you how many people I've treated over the years who have injured their spines due to faulty sports equipment.

Take the time to gently warm up prior to strenuous activity, and as always, remain hydrated throughout the activity.

As a basic rule, carb up prior to your activity to have ample ready-energy while you play, and follow up with a higher protein meal immediately after so your body can use the available amino acids to repair muscles after you finish.

Part III: All right, now what?
Onward and Upward!

So, we've covered quite a lot of ground up to this point. We've talked about your sleep, wake time, fun in bed, your commute, your psyche, your workplace, your kitchen, your kids, and a whole bunch of other things- all of which are designed to get you to the goal of a life free from back pain. It's a lot to absorb. As you embark on this journey towards a pain-free lifestyle, I encourage you to pause for a moment and ask the question you should be asking *every single day for the rest of your life*: **What will you do for your back today?**

Right now, think back through all of the things we've covered so far, and choose three things you'd like to do as soon as possible. I'll just sit here and check my email for few minutes while you think about it....

1)_____

2)_____

3)_____

Now take a look at the three you chose. Do they all apply to one area of your life? Are they all workplace related? Are they all in your kitchen? Or perhaps you chose some modifications in different areas of your life? Do you remember earlier when I said that success leaves clues? Here is where you get your first clues: Your body knows what it needs, and based upon your first choices of anatomic bombs to address- you now have a pretty good idea of where to start off on this journey of healing. If it was your workplace or kitchen that was the first place your head took you- that's where you should start. If you chose several diffuse, unrelated areas, then you are going to have to spend a little time trying some of these suggestions, and then following up and looking for even more clues. Most people will start to see patterns over time, and these patterns will help you to improve and refine your plan. Again, the key thing here is to be committed to making changes, and to *know* that these changes are leading you toward your desired outcome- to rid yourself of back and neck pain *forever*.

Interestingly, most patients I've worked with do wind up with a more varied list for the first few things they choose to address. I feel like there are two primary reasons for this. First, as I've said over and over, your back pain is most certainly being caused by a whole host of contributing factors from various areas of your life. Secondly, if you were to identify one area, such as your kitchen, as the source of your pain, you've probably given some thought to the ergonomics of that area already. In the spirit of the cumulative nature of the causes of back and neck pain, I thought this would be a great place to share with you my *Super Double Secret Top Fifteen List for Reducing Back and Neck Pain (It used to be a top ten list- but now its new and improved with five wonderful new tips!)*. This list represents the fifteen modifications, which I have clinically seen to be the most effective across the broadest cross section of patients I have cared for over the years. It has been modified and enhanced since my last book- so if you are familiar with that list you should probably take a moment to read this new and improved list. You've already seen most of these suggestions in the different sections of the book- this list is designed to simply give you a quick checklist of those that, statistically speaking, may give you the biggest 'bang for your back.' Let's say you are a total slacker. Somehow you made it through to this point in my book. You just cannot see yourself going to the trouble to take the steps to get pain out of your life. If you do absolutely *nothing* else in this book, **do these:**

Fifteen Surefire Tips for Relieving Back Pain:

1. **Buy a cordless headset for your telephone or mobile phone.** Not cradling the handset between your shoulder and ear will go farther than almost anything else you can do in your daily life to reduce neck discomfort.

2. **If you *carry a briefcase, purse, or book bag, go through the contents and see what you can do to lighten its weight.*** Do you actually need all of the items, or are you just carrying them due to habit? Also, shop for a lightweight bag- some handbags and briefcases weigh a ton *empty.*

3. ***If you carry one of these bags, or a child, or groceries, or anything on a regular basis, try to alternate sides.*** This will take some of the strain off of overused muscles and joints, and give you the chance to strengthen the less favored side.

4. ***If you sit for longer than forty-five minutes to an hour at a time, stand up and stretch your legs and lower back.*** As I described earlier, reach up to the sky with your arms, and move your neck throughout its entire range of motion in all directions. Remember, you weren't designed to sit nearly as much as you probably do.

5. ***If you have more than five minutes to spare- take a coffee break walk.*** This is not intended to replace any of your cardiovascular exercise, but rather, to get you up and moving. This will help prevent joint stiffness, get your blood flowing, clear

your head and get some air into your lungs.

6. ***Make sure your computer monitor, keyboard and mouse are in the proper location.*** If you sit and stare at a computer monitor for much of the day, be sure to move your head into different positions periodically to avoid getting 'stuck.'

7. I know I've mentioned this about a thousand times, but ***several times throughout your day, take a moment for 3-4 deep cleansing breaths.***

8. ***Try to maintain your body weight within 5-7 percent of your optimal body mass index*** (you can find your optimal BMI online or in countless references.)

9. ***Use proper lifting technique when picking up heavy objects, your children, or any other items you need to carry.*** While you are

carrying them, keep the bulk of their mass close to your center of gravity (for example, carry your children on your hip). Again- make an effort to change sides frequently.

10. ***Get cardiovascular exercise at least four times a week.*** Try to vary the activity regularly in order to keep your body guessing, and take advantage of the benefits of cross training.

11. ***Get regular hydration.*** I originally included this with the exercise tip above, but I wanted to stress that this should happen *all day long*. Being properly hydrated helps to lubricate your joints, forces you to get up from a seated position regularly, and keeps you from feeling too hungry- which can help to manage your weight more effectively.

12. ***Get regular sleep.*** Quantity is not nearly as important as quality and regularity. While I don't

recommend walking around sleep deprived, it is important to remember that a few hours of good deep sleep can be much more beneficial than a whole night of restless, shallow sleep.

13. ***Take a few minutes to slowly wake up, and do a brief morning stretch as I described earlier.*** Awakening gently can set the tone for your entire day.

14. ***Break up household tasks, such as dusting or vacuuming, into smaller, more manageable blocks.*** Maybe do one or two rooms a day rather than trying to conquer the whole house once a week.

15. ***Set aside a portion of every day to relax and unwind.*** Use this time to take a few of our oft-mentioned deep cleansing breaths and recharge. Reflect upon your day and find a way to achieve your most calm state, even if only for a few moments.

Again, quality over quantity. Use this time to acknowledge the times you haven't been in as much pain today, or perhaps when it was not as severe as at other times.

Congratulations!

It borders on tragic that so many people choose to live with back & neck pain. The folks who accept the pain and believe they have no control over it write their own epitaph (Here lies a dude with back pain- lying down, because he couldn't find another comfortable position...). What the hell is the matter with these people?!?! *Congratulations! You have just taken what might be your first action steps towards living a pain free lifestyle.* As you slowly and methodically apply some of your newfound knowledge, you may notice that you will start to see the world around you in a different way: you will be able to recognize the anatomic bombs around you without someone like me guiding you. I often cite the slogan of a retail chain that states 'An educated consumer is our best customer.' From my standpoint, an educated patient is *my* best customer. One of the reasons people do wind up back in the doctor's office over and over again, is because their lifestyle sends them down the same path over and over again. You are now the educated consumer. You are the guru. You know how to change your path, and go down the one that will keep you pain free.

Having the knowledge and then actually *using it* are completely different things. You don't need me to tell you that none of this will matter if you don't do something. Albert Einstein once said "Nothing happens unless something moves." Now is your time to *get moving*. Back pain frequently sticks around because of things that you are doing- possibly things you are doing *every single day*. Here is where I call upon you once again- take a positive step *every single day*. Remember to begin each day by answering the question *"What will I do for my back today?"* End each day by answering the question *"What did I do for my back today?"* When you begin to answer those questions every day with honest, concrete responses, you will know that the pain has stopped controlling you- but rather you are the one who is in control.

Be well!

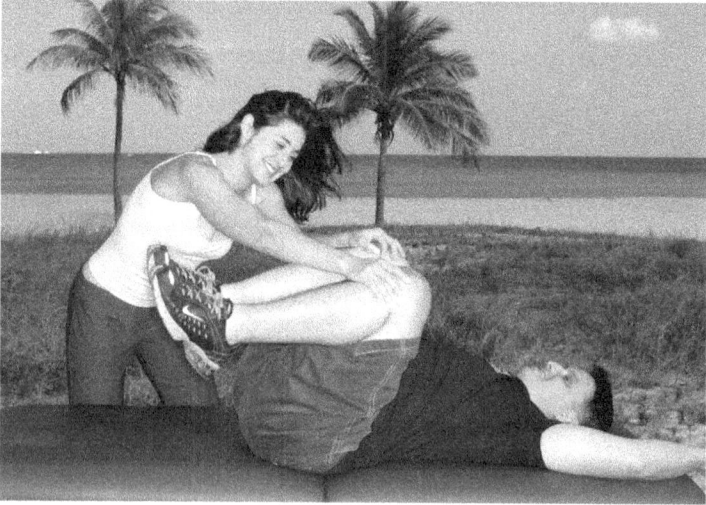

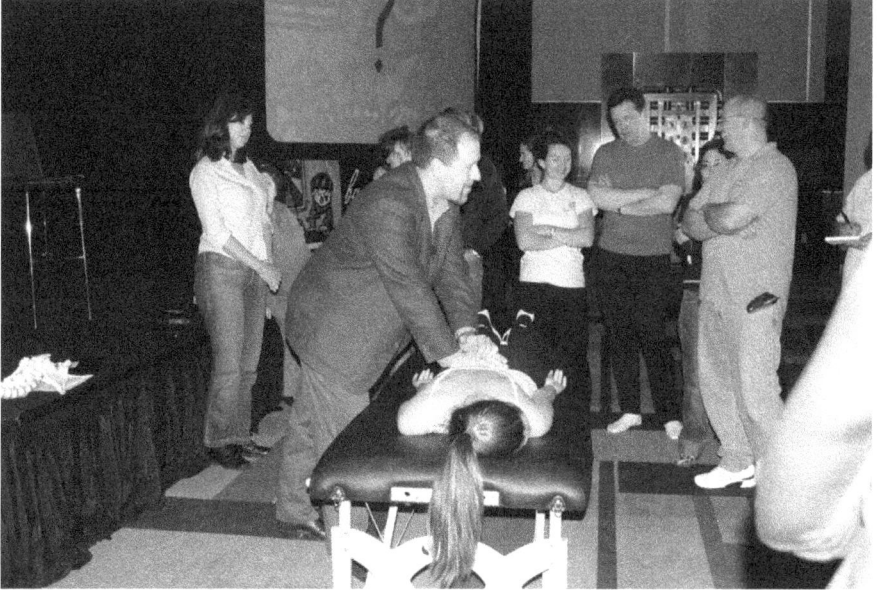

Scene from another Back Together Live seminar.

About the Author

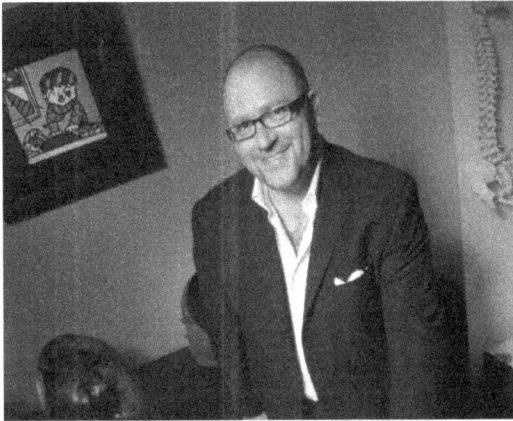

Dr. Andrew Kirschner is a board certified physician and Assistant Clinical Professor at the Philadelphia College of Osteopathic Medicine. He teaches his techniques both to clinicians and to laypersons in his *Back Together* live seminars.

For over 15 years, professional athletes and the physically challenged, adolescents and the elderly have all benefitted from Dr. Kirschner's, unique approach to back & neck pain. He has been featured in many national publications including Martha Stewart Living, Andrew Weil's Self-Healing, and Psychology Today. He has been a regular guest on Whole Living Radio and the Veria Network.

Dr. Kirschner maintains a private practice in Bala Cynwyd, PA and a peak performance consultancy in Miami, FL. He lives with his wife Donna and their two daughters. His loves playing and composing for the piano, mountain biking, drawing and vintage auto mechanics. You can reach him through his website, BackTogetherCentral.com

Oh, and before I forget- here is a form you can use for tracking your progress. You can fill these in using a table format, and track how your pain responds to any type of variable you choose: Lifestyle modifications, activities, sleep, etc... Like I said earlier, success and failure both leave clues. Here is one way to gather and analyze these clues.

Subjective Pain Analysis (SPA)

Date:

Head:

Neck:

Mid back:

Low back:

Sciatic:

Upper extremity R:

Upper extremity L:

Lower extremity R:

Lower extremity L:

I love to hear from readers!

Please send any of your questions or comments to:

Info@backtogether.org

www.ingramcontent.com/pod-product-compliance
Lightning Source LLC
Chambersburg PA
CBHW021618270326
41931CB00008B/757